WHY WE NEED TO DETOX

The Benefits of Detoxing Your Body to
Reduce Gut Inflammation, Bloating, and
Brain Fog

SACHA LUCAS

MagletPublishing

ISBN: 978-1-7399248-3-6

Contents

Introduction

Starting Your Detox Journey

Incorporating detoxification into your life is simple, effective, and safe. Like beginning any journey, it requires planning, organization, and a lot of determination, but the pay off when you reach your destination is worth the effort. You can live a happier, healthier, pain-free life by controlling what you eat and removing the toxins from your system.

A Food Cleanse Experience

Detoxification is an experience for anyone who wants to learn how to better take care of their body but is held back by being too busy or simply not knowing where to begin. If you're looking for guidance to get you started on your detoxification journey, you're in the right place.

There is a vast array of symptoms that might encourage you to take up detoxification. This includes, but isn't limited to, things like bloating, constipation or poor bowel movements; fatigue and poor sleeping patterns; migraines or headaches; indigestion and acid reflux; obesity and food cravings. These symptoms can be made even worse by day-to-day experiences and choices such as prescribed medications, high cholesterol, food intolerances, caffeine consumption, and smoking. It's quite the list, and these symptoms can be extraordinarily frustrating.

The Detoxification Journey is an Opportunity to Heal and Repair Your Body

How do you make sure that the poisons and toxins from your food, water, air, and environment are fully eliminated from your body? Well, you need to let your body metabolize all these harmful substances into being less toxic and more easily excreted. That's exactly what detoxification is designed to do.

When you stick to your detox plan, you can become a healthier, happier person with higher energy levels, improved immunity, and improved digestion. You'll even feel lighter, have a clearer mind, and will find better control over your food intolerances and cravings. Who wouldn't want to have all that?

This journey provides an opportunity to learn how you can truly take care of yourself. Smart detoxification is not a dangerous body cleanse, but a smarter approach to health through eating the right foods and improving your overall lifestyle. You can reach your goals, and you can be the best version of yourself.

Let's get started on this wonderful journey together!

What is Detox? Is it for Me?

To many people, the detox process is like a much-needed vacation for the body. Those lucky ones have higher energy, more balanced blood sugar, are able to sleep better, and feel like they're on cloud nine! But for others, detoxing can mean that brain fog starts to settle in like rough weather. They start to feel irritable, moody, weak, hungry, and sometimes have symptoms like they're suffering from the flu. For some others, hyper-sensitivity takes them over, making it extremely challenging for them to follow through with the detoxification program, especially those in which they need herbal support.

So, why is there a difference? Why do some people get to feel great when they go through this process while the rest do not? It all depends on the defense mechanism of their body and how it eliminates the toxins consumed in day-to-day life.

Detoxification, or detox, is a fancy name for selecting foods and other lifestyle changes to help the body's cleansing routine flourish. It can work wonders, but most people go about it in the wrong way. As a result, they feel terrible and give up before reaching the reward of positive results at the end. How can we control this process and reach our goals?

If we consider all the toxins that we absorb from our food, water, and even the air we breathe, it makes sense we would want to remove them as fast as possible.

But such an approach almost always backfires. Most of us have been building up these toxins for years, so we can't get rid of them all at once without feeling awful as they move through our bodies. Instead, we need to learn to support our body's natural systems to eliminate the unhealthy waste products. Our bodies are well designed to deal with toxins but can accomplish it even more efficiently when we're doing the right things to prevent more build up and ease the flow of toxins through these systems.

If it helps, think of your body as a humongous city in which every house is a cell. Imagine what would happen if the homeowner takes the garbage out of the house every day, but the trash never gets taken from the street? It would definitely pile up and lead to problems.

The same thing happens to our bodies. Through detoxification you can increase the rate of toxins being removed from your cells and out of your body. But unless you strengthen the elimination systems those toxins can't be properly removed and will build up around your cells. This could lead to worsening the symptoms that you're working to improve.

For the same reason, it's crucial for you to have an effective routine that starts your detox journey with drainage.

In the following chapters, you will learn how your body detoxes naturally and how the drainage pathways open up to let the toxins out of your body.

How Does Your Body Detox?

When we hear the word detoxification, we might think of pills and shakes and other nutritional supplements that force the water and toxins out of the body. In reality detoxification refers to the process of removing toxins through natural body systems run by a healthy metabolism. I wish the supplement and wellness industries would acknowledge that detoxification is something our bodies already do! Detoxification is a process that our body is very good at, involving all our organs and the digestive, urinary, cardiovascular, respiratory, and lymphatic systems. But sometimes these systems need more support to function at their best.

Let's talk a little about these systems and how they're involved in detoxification.

Skin

The largest organ in your body is the skin, which is covered by tiny openings called pores. Your skin eliminates toxins through those pores in sweat and body oils. When you perspire, your body eliminates toxins, including heavy metals, such as mercury, lead, arsenic, and cadmium. To support your skin's natural detoxification process, you need to keep the skin clean so the pores aren't clogged. Regular exercise is also important both for your metabolism and the healthy movement of perspiration. Stay well hydrated too and sweat it out!

Kidneys and Urinary System

The primary function of your kidneys is to eliminate waste, toxins, and excess water that move through your circulatory system. The kidneys extract these products and turn them into urine. To carry this process out effectively, your kidneys must be supported by good hydration, provided when you drink sufficient water, and by eating a good, healthy diet that is filled with whole, fresh foods. Removing foods from your diet that are highly processed and that contain added sodium and chemicals is great for kidney function.

Digestive System

The function of the colon is to move waste products from the body, so it's clear that its role in eliminating toxins from the body is critical. This has led to the idea of a "colon cleanse" as a popular method for detoxing. However, the belief that fecal matter can be lodged in your colon and be absorbed back into your bloodstream is not true. Your digestive tract consists of a cell lining that regenerates constantly and makes this idea impossible. However, slow moving fecal matter is a problem, and you do need good digestion in order to properly support the process of elimination. You can protect good gut health by consuming food rich in fiber, prebiotics, and probiotics.

For all these three mechanisms to function efficiently, ensure that you feed your body with the right kind of nutrients, give it sufficient rest, and drink plenty of water. When you stay properly hydrated, sweat regularly, and poop normally, you are enabling the elimination pathways of your body to do their jobs effectively.

The Liver

Your liver acts as the detoxification hub in your body. It's a powerhouse when it comes to removing toxins from the body. This large organ deals with toxins consumed in foods, such as caffeine and alcohol. But it also removes excess hormones, like estrogen, and medicines, like antibiotics. Many of the toxins the liver removes are naturally produced. But your lifestyle, including diet, sleeping routine, medication overuse, smoking, and environment, puts additional stress on this powerhouse. It's vital that we give our liver the support it requires.

How to Support the Natural Detox Pathways of Your Body

Now that we've identified some of the systems and organs that are responsible for natural detoxification, what can you do to support these systems? Let's consider a few ideas that you can easily implement and might not have considered.

- Drinking enough water: It's essential to consume plenty of water throughout the day in order to keep your body hydrated. We're often encouraged to drink eight eight-ounce glasses of water a day, and that's a good rule of thumb. But in reality, everyone has slightly different hydration needs. To determine your own starting place for how much water you need to drink each day, use this simple formula: divide your body weight (in pounds) by 2 to get the number of ounces you should drink every day. Remember this is a rough guide.

Example:

170 lbs ÷ 2 = 85 ounces
85 ounces = 10.6 cups or 2.4 liters of water

Those who exercise regularly or who are otherwise very active in their daily life will need additional water beyond this starting amount. Furthermore, if you consume caffeinated or alcoholic beverages, you need to increase your water consumption.

- Taking deep breaths: The lungs are detox organs as well, as they remove carbon dioxide and other waste gases from our bodies. When the lungs are working well, they ensure oxygen circulates throughout the body, giving strength to your cells and reducing stress. That's why deep breathing is an effective remedy for anxiety. So, take a few deep breaths and exhale completely in between your tasks or whenever you feel overwhelmed, and make sure you feel your rib cage expanding and contracting.
- Moving your body: When you get up and get moving, it supports literally every system in your body through increased blood flow and better oxygenation. What's more, if you lead a sedentary lifestyle, lymphatic fluid can build up and cause swelling and joint pain. Even gentle exercise can help to get everything moving for better detox and flexibility.
- Visiting an infrared sauna: If you can, aim to have a few sessions of infrared sauna a month to promote efficient detoxification. The benefits of

this type of sauna include increased sweat production, reduced inflammation, relaxed muscles, and better circulation.

- Supporting your gut health: You can support good health in your gut by consuming a diet that is rich in probiotics, prebiotics, fiber, fermented vegetables, collagen, and bone broth. When your intestines are functioning at their optimum, they are better able to get rid of the waste from your body.

How are Your Gut and Mind Connected?

When we talk about detoxification, one of the issues we want to address is how detox can help with not only your physical health but your mental health as well. You might not realize it, but these things are connected! In the same way that your emotional state can give you the sensation of butterflies in your stomach or make you shake, the food you eat, and how your body deals with it, has a direct effect on your mental state.

Gut-Brain Axis

The gut-brain axis is a system of two-way communication between your stomach and brain. It maintains your body's homeostasis, which is a state of stable functioning. The gut-brain axis comprises:

- Brain
- Enteric nervous system or nerves surrounding your gut
- Vagus nerve

7

- Hormones like serotonin
- Gut bacteria

Effect of Gut on Brain

Just like your brain affects the operation of your gut, your gut health has an impact on your brain and mental health too. When there is an unusual distribution of bacteria inside your gut or a build-up of toxins, it can complicate conditions such as schizophrenia and spectrum disorders.

A good detox diet can help you achieve and maintain a balance between your gut and mental health and, with guidance from a medical professional, help prevent or improve these disorders.

What Foods Help the Gut-Brain Axis?

There are a few food groups that are particularly beneficial to your gut-brain axis.

- Omega-3 fatty acids: Omega-3 fatty acids are found in fish oils and some plant-based oils. However, they are also found in the human brain. These fatty acids assist in increasing gut bacteria which, in turn, reduces the risk of several brain disorders.
- High-fiber foods: The prebiotic fibers that are good for the gut are found in nuts, whole grains, seeds, vegetables, and fruits. They also help in lowering stress hormones.
- Fermented foods: Yogurt, cheese, sauerkraut, and kefir contain healthy microbes, like the lactic acid

bacteria. These fermented foods also help to improve brain activity.

- Tryptophan-rich foods: Tryptophan is a type of amino acid that gets converted into serotonin, a neurotransmitter. Tryptophan is found in cheese, eggs, and turkey.
- Polyphenol-rich foods: Coffee, green tea, cocoa, and olive oil contain polyphenols. These are plant chemicals that get digested by gut bacteria. Polyphenols are compounds that support healthy gut bacteria and enhanced cognition.

So you see that your body and mind are amazing machines with all the tools they need for effective detoxification. We've touched briefly on supporting your body's natural detoxification abilities and your mental health, but let's dig deeper.

What is a Detox Diet?

Typically, detox diets are short-term eating plans that are designed to force the elimination of toxins from the body.

Most detox diets consist of a fasting period followed by a strict eating regime of fruits, fruit juices, vegetables, and lots of water. Often these diets will also include teas, supplements, herbs, and enemas or colon cleanses.

This type of detox diet helps by:

- Promoting elimination of toxins via urine, sweat, and feces
- Resting your organs through fasting

- Improving blood circulation
- Stimulating the liver
- Replenishing your body with healthy nutrients

When applied correctly, this detoxing plan can ease bloating, inflammation, allergies, chronic fatigue, obesity, autoimmune diseases, and digestive tract issues.

Juice Detoxes

As discussed, most detox diets are designed to eliminate harmful chemicals and toxins in the body by stimulating natural elimination. These plans can also act as a kind of 'reset' for the body after a prolonged period of consuming excess processed foods. Many people turn to detoxing following holidays, for example.

We mentioned eating plenty of fruits and vegetables, but some detoxification eating patterns will recommend consuming nothing but juice for three to five days, restricting calorie consumption along with proteins, fats, and most carbohydrates.

Here are some tips to make the most of this type of scheme:

- Opt for herbal teas over caffeinated teas. When you consume low-caffeine or caffeine-free teas, like parsley, ginger, or dandelion root, it creates less stress on your liver, making for a healthy and light detox for your body. You can consume these teas twice a day, once before breakfast and once before dinner. This will make it easier for your digestive system and assist in the functioning of your liver and kidneys as well.

- As always, it's important to stay hydrated. When you drink plenty of water during the day, you're enabling your body's detox systems to flush out the toxins. It also helps to enhance the functioning of your internal organs and is important for the health of your skin. Always consume a minimum of two liters of water a day to detox your body in the simplest, most natural way.

Difference Between Detox and Cleansing

There are several differences between a detox and a cleanse, but people often use the terms interchangeably, especially on the internet where the amount of information you find is sometimes conflicting and can be overwhelming. This makes it even more confusing when we're looking for a healthy way to break a weight-loss plateau or get back on track after a vacation or holiday.

So, let's take a look at these two terms, break down the key differences between them, and consider the pros and cons of each.

Cleanse

When we talk about a body cleanse, think of your gut health. If you feel constipated or bloated, you might need to cleanse your digestive tract. As discussed earlier, matter in your digestive tract cannot be reabsorbed into your body, however, it can move slowly and thereby cause discomfort and sluggishness. The first step in a cleanse is to eliminate foods that are harder on the digestive system. For most people, this will include refined sugars, caffeinated products, soy, gluten, eggs, dairy products, processed foods, red meat, and alcohol. As you remove these foods from your diet and replace them with healthier options like fruit, vegetables and high-quality grains, it facilitates the work of your digestive tract and helps move fecal matter through while at the same time encouraging the growth of healthy gut bacteria.

The primary goal of a body cleanse is to give your digestive system a rest, help combat bloating, and support regular bowel movements.

Detox

Detox, on the other hand, is focused on helping to improve your kidney and liver health. The kidneys and liver work with the other organs of your body to naturally eliminate toxins. However, they may well need a little boost, too, sometimes. Just like cleansing, you begin detoxing by removing unhealthy foods and those that encourage a buildup of waste, such as alcohol, processed foods, and sugars. Once you eliminate these items, you feed the body with juice and water to help flush out any remaining toxins. Then you can reintroduce foods that help in strengthening your kidney and liver functions, such as garlic, pineapple, lemon, ginger, and kale.

The biggest advantage of detoxification is that it helps your organs to release toxins, neutralize them, and eliminate them in a way that is restorative on a deep cellular level. The thorough hydration achieved through detox doesn't only relieve bloating and discomfort, but it also revitalizes and restores your system from the inside out.

Before you opt for a detox or cleanse, you should consider your personal health conditions and may want to talk to your doctor. Some medical conditions preclude a detox diet or may require that you modify your detox. Always be sure to listen to your body, drink plenty of water, get sufficient sleep, and get some exercise.

Types of Detoxes

Detox diets are characterized by short-term changes in your day-to-day eating patterns by removing most foods and consuming fruits, vegetables, juice and water. This process helps by removing toxins that have built up in your body. This type of eating plan also aims to boost immunity, increase energy, and improve blood circulation.

Detox programs come with several benefits, the greatest of which is the improvement in your eating habits and your approach towards food overall. These diets are not just meant to bring about changes physically, but mentally as well by enhancing your clarity and focus.

Other aspects of a detox diet may include:

- Fasting
- Eating only specific foods
- Drinking only juices or other restricted beverages
- Consuming herbs and herbal teas
- Cleansing the colon with laxatives, enemas, or colon hydrotherapy
- Using a sauna
- Using dietary supplements or other commercial products
- Reducing environmental exposure

Liver Cleanse

Your liver is the focus of most detox diets, since it collects most toxins from what you eat and drink. You can detox your liver by consuming lemons, carrots, beetroots, limes, and celery. Spices, such as cumin, curry, and turmeric assist in detoxifying the liver as well. Avoid soda — both diet and full sugar — coffee and caffeinated tea when you want to detox your liver. Instead, opt for apple juice or, the best of all, pure water.

Sugar Detoxification

Another classic focus for a detox is sugar, also called a candida cleanse. The aim of this process is to get rid of all foods that contain sugar and promote candida. On this diet, you avoid all kinds of refined foods and the ones that contain added sweeteners and sugars. You must avoid yeast as well, so you need to stay away from most bread, cheese, alcohol, dried fruit, mushrooms, pickles, and soy sauce.

Colon Cleanse

As we have already seen, the colon is another organ where toxins can build up. When you follow a detox diet for your colon, you consume distilled water, raw, unfiltered apple cider vinegar, probiotics, and aloe vera.

Liquid Cleanse

As the name suggests, this diet is based on consuming only liquids. It works well for people who find the restrictions of only fruit juice and water too extreme or who may feel run down from getting insufficient calories. When following a liquid cleanse, you would be consuming soups, juices, smoothies, flax, coconut, coconut water, pumpkin, and hemp seed oil, apart from drinking plenty of water.

Alkaline Cleanse

An alkaline cleanse depends on consuming raw vegetables, fruit, seeds, and nuts as well as increasing your water consumption. The purpose is to detoxify your entire body, from your liver to your colon. It offers the added benefit of already consisting of alkaline food, so there is no further need for food alkalization, which is a common in many modern diets.

Ayurvedic Cleanse

Based on ancient whole-body healing principles, the Ayurvedic cleanse is designed to cleanse your body entirely and provide relief to your digestive system. It focuses on consuming cooked vegetables, spices, rice, and mung beans.

You can also enhance the diet by eating cleansing herbs, such as dandelion, cilantro, alfalfa, or milk thistle.

Cleansing Spices

Adding herbs and spices to your cleanse can be very effective. It also brings flavor to a diet that can be bland as it's often without much variety. Herbs and spices can be important for your good health in general, even when you aren't cleansing or detoxing. Choose ginger, turmeric, oregano, parsley, rosemary, cloves, cumin, cinnamon, cayenne pepper, and fenugreek, since they complement your meals and help to detoxify your body.

Why Should You Choose a Detox Diet?

As discussed earlier, following a detox diet has many benefits, both physical and mental. It not only cleanses your body to remove toxins, but also supports your mental health. Detox brings about a sense of peace, calm, and freshness within your body, and makes you feel energized and rejuvenated.

Many cultures encourage fasting in order to bring about targeted changes in the body to provide a feeling of serenity while building discipline. So the idea of fasting or limiting diets to certain foods is not some newfangled, new-age fad.

At one time, detox diets were mostly used to target weight loss. However, as more and more people have tried such diets, we have learned how beneficial it is to decrease the consumption of coffee, alcohol, and other foods. And we have discovered how detoxing can help us overcome health issues and improving our eating habits.

Benefits of a Detox Diet

There are many tangible advantages to following a detox diet. These benefits include:

- Healthy hair and skin

When you remove toxins from your body and are properly hydrated, your skin becomes firmer, fuller, and healthier. It also reduces acne and encourages clear skin while removing some visible signs of aging.

Detox diets also leave your hair shinier, healthier, and stronger. Toxins building up in your hair follicles prevent your hair from growing, making it dull, brittle, and lifeless. When the build up is removed from your follicles, healthy hair growth is the result.

- Weight loss and a stronger digestive system

The removal of unnecessary waste from your body enables vitamins and nutrients to be more readily absorbed into your body. Also, these diets help to speed up your metabolism, which leads to easier long-term weight management.

- Boosted immune system

Since greater amounts of minerals and vitamins are absorbed into your body, your vital organs are healthier, boosting your immunity. Cleanses also remove harmful bacteria from your body and encourage the growth of healthy gut bacteria.

• Improved mental health

Detox diets help you have better focus, clarity, and sleep. For these reasons, they play a crucial role in improving your psychological and emotional well-being.

• Added antioxidants

Fruit contains several antioxidant-rich nutrients, like vitamins A, B, C and E, so a detox diet helps increase the antioxidant levels in your body. An eating plan that focuses on juice and water also improves the circulation of blood with proper hydration.

• Mindful eating

Irrespective of the cleansing and additional hydration, you will also experience an improved relationship with the food you consume. This is because you will be mindful of the kind of food you put into your body.

Participating in a detox diet certainly helps you to build a healthier lifestyle, and you start to appreciate your body more. You become more critical of what you eat since you are aware of the effects it will have on your body. This can lead to a healthier balance in your life.

Begin Your Detox Journey

We've learned what a detox diet is, why it's important, and why you would benefit from it. Now, let us discuss how to start.

- The very first thing you might want to do is consult your doctor, nutritionist, or other healthcare professional. You need to ensure that there will be no detrimental effects on your body when you begin.
- Prepare yourself to give up alcohol, coffee, black tea, and cold, flavored drinks. Replace them with water, lemon water, or herbal teas.
- Select a detox diet that best suits your needs. This might vary from one person to another, depending on your body's needs and overall calorie intake.
- When toxins are being flushed from your body in the initial stages, you might experience symptoms like headache, vomiting, and nausea. These can also be the result of eliminating chemicals like caffeine from your diet. You must be prepared for these situations and push through them to get to the results you desire.
- Be sure to plan your detox diet in such a way that you're still consuming the calories and nutrients your body needs. A pure detox diet does not include the proteins or carbohydrates of a typical healthy, balanced diet. That's why these diets should be used for a limited time. You must make sure that your body gets proper nutrition in a healthier manner.
- Avoid heavy exercising when you are on your detox diet. You need to get your body moving to encourage the efficient removal of toxins, but heavy exercise during periods where you're consuming fewer calories, fats, proteins, and carbohydrates can be tiring or even dangerous.

- During the course of the diet your tongue might feel like it's covered in a coating. You can try chewing sugar-free gum, sucking on mints or using a tongue scraper to get rid of the bacteria layer.
- If you wish to improve your gut health, try consuming fruits and vegetables that are particularly rich in fiber, like beans, cruciferous vegetables, apples and berries.
- Once your detox diet is over, make sure to re-introduce solid foods in your diet slowly. Your digestive system will be disrupted if you suddenly start to eat solid food after several days of liquid or primarily liquid consumption.

For a Juice Diet

- Focus on using organic vegetables and fruits.
- Opt for making your own juices at home rather than purchasing them pre-packaged since those often contain excess sugar and preservatives. This definitely goes against the purpose of a detox diet.
- Use whole fruits as much as possible when you are juicing, which includes the peels as long as they are not excessively bitter. The peels of fruits and vegetables contain minerals and nutrients that are enormously beneficial for your body.
- Make sure you consume the juice immediately after you make it. It's not recommended to store it and have it later.
- Include fruits that have a lower glycemic index, meaning those that contain less natural sugar. You might not particularly like how certain green

vegetables taste, but those are going to be the ones that contain the maximum nutrients.

- You can try enhancing the flavor and consistency of your juice by adding some herbs and spices.
- Ensure that you are fully hydrated throughout your juice diet. Just drinking juice at mealtimes will not provide enough fluid for your body while it's removing toxins. You will also need to drink plenty of fresh water.

The Detox Process

I could make a very long list of the different fancy names of the so-called detoxes that have gained popularity in the last few years. All of these diets claim to improve your health and facilitate weight loss, often in some miraculous manner! But do these diets and fads actually help to detox your body? To answer that question, we let's delve deeper into natural detoxification.

The Natural Detoxification Process of the Body

Yes, it's true that our body can and does detoxify itself. We have systems that maintain efficient housekeeping to remove toxins, chemicals, and non-usable substances that enter our bodies. So, how do these processes work? We've touched on this before, but let's go a little further.

Antibodies and Enzymes

Enzymes are proteins with the function of breaking down larger molecules into smaller, functional substances that our body puts to use. For instance, we have enzymes that help break down large proteins into smaller molecules called amino acids. These amino acids are useful in building muscle tissue. When there is a molecule intake that the enzyme does not recognize, such as a foreign chemical, for example, it gets absorbed fully instead of broken down. When the body doesn't recognize a substance, the immune system reacts by producing antibodies. These antibodies come to the rescue and figure out what to do with the foreign substance, usually excreting it back into the bloodstream or storing it within fat cells until it can be removed.

Fat Cell Storage

When our immune system works at its best and there are not many external chemicals that it has to deal with, the antibodies—along with several other nutrients—mix the introduced chemical up with other substances to be discarded from the body. In case where the immune system is overworked, or if there are several chemicals coming in, antibodies shuttle them into triglycerides or fat cells. These fat cells are then safely stored in the body without causing any harm. Of course, the downside of this is that we are storing more and more fat cells to hold foreign substances that are introduced.

Phase 1 Detox

For antibodies to pack up toxins and chemicals to eliminate them or release them from triglycerides, specific nutrients need to be present in your body in large amounts. These nutrients are B vitamins, the antioxidant vitamins C and E, the fat-soluble vitamins A and D, calcium, milk thistle, and glutathione. The sources of these nutrients include bright-colored fruits and vegetables, nuts, seeds, and wild fish. When there are not enough of these nutrients in your body and toxins are not released, it can adversely affect the body in the form of organ tissue damage or even lead to some cancers in cases where the retained chemicals are carcinogenic.

Phase 2 Detox

When your body is healthy, there are plenty of nutrients from phase 1 circulating in your bloodstream. Your body is ready to pack up the toxins and chemicals for elimination. These chemicals need to move through the body to get eliminated without creating any damage along the way. To enable this to happen, specific amino acids, such as taurine, glycine, sulfur, glutamine, and cysteine are required. We obtain these amino acids from seeds, nuts, wild fish, and vegetables like onions, cauliflower, and broccoli. When our body is low on these phase 2 nutrients, all these chemicals and toxins get sent right back into our bloodstream!

Elimination

If we assume that we have all the right nutrients and our immune system is working at its best, all that's left is the elimination of these toxins. Elimination occurs through sweat, urine, feces, and even our breath. But any impedi-ment to one or more of these functions can hinder our body's ability to flush out the unwanted waste. For example, if our kidneys do not function properly, or we're constipated, or even if we use antiperspirants every day to block our armpits producing sweat, we might not be eliminating as many toxins as we should be. So, what happens to these toxins? Again, they head straight back to your bloodstream!

How to Support a Healthy Detox

Fortunately, there's a lot that you can do to enable your detox pathways to open up naturally. Take a look at the phases of detox above and then consider how you can support each step.

- The first step is to limit the intake of chemicals and toxins in the first place. Opt for organic produce and purchase fewer food items packaged in plastic.
- Eat less processed food and more whole foods.
- Consume more plants and foods that are rich in the nutrients that target your detox pathways.
- If you are constipated, increase your intake of water and fiber, and make sure to stretch and exercise.
- Exercise till you sweat a few days a week.
- Consume water like it's your job!

Key Takeaways

So, we've learned what a detox diet is and some of the many different types you might choose, according to your body's needs. We also determined that detox is a short-term plan to help eliminate toxins and harmful chemicals from your body.

Of course, detoxing will assist your body to deal with several different issues. But why should you choose detox? In the next chapter we'll look at the different kinds of toxins that need to be cleansed and how they harmful to our bodies.

2

Body Toxins

The word "toxin" may sound extreme and like some kind of invention of the modern era, but in fact the absorption of toxins from food and the environment has been an issue for hundreds of years. Of course, it does tend to align more readily with modernization and our advanced, "civilized" lifestyles, but as an example, 200 years ago, doctors frequently diagnosed "mad hatter disease" in people who worked in the hat making industry. Although this disease sounds like a fairytale, it was actually the result of mercury poisoning from the materials in the hats. In another example, some believe that toxins from lead water pipes were a significant cause of the decline of the Roman Empire.

Over time it became accepted in the medical field that illness from toxins could be linked to occupation. People who performed certain tasks were known to be at risk, such as coal miners who inhaled toxic coal dust. At that time, doctors did not consider that the rest of the population could be at risk as well, but the modern proliferation of industrial activities and products is causing this perspective to shift. A great deal of modern research is focused on understanding how toxins affect all humans. The more I read about toxins and how they affect us, the more I'm convinced that what we see is just the tip of a huge iceberg.

How Toxins Damage Our Bodies

In general terms, there are eight different ways in which toxins damage our bodies.

Poison Enzymes and Inhibit their Functioning

Our bodies are engines that run on enzymes, proteins that break up and create molecules. Each physiological function in our body relies on enzymes for producing energy, manufacturing molecules, and forming cell structures. Toxins damage these enzymes and thereby inhibit our bodily functions, including the production of hemoglobin in our blood. This damage also lowers the body's capacity to avoid free-radical damage that leads to premature aging and some cancers.

Weaken Bones

We need to maintain a healthy bone mass to stay mobile. When toxins displace the calcium in our bones, our skeletal structures get weaker. As if that wasn't bad enough, this bone loss releases additional toxins that then circulate throughout the body.

Damage Our Organs

Toxins can damage all of our bodily organs and systems. If your kidneys, liver, and digestive tract become toxic they can no longer eliminate waste, and the entire natural detoxification system is slowed or stopped altogether.

Damage DNA

Some commonly used, improperly detoxified substances such as estrogen, phthalates, pesticides and products that contain benzene can actually harm our DNA. This injury can lead to degeneration and premature aging. Furthermore, these problems can be passed to children in pregnant women.

Modify Gene Expression

Our genes naturally switch on and off to adapt to the changes our body goes through as it ages as well as in response to our environment. However, several toxins either suppress or activate our genes in an unhealthy manner.

Damage Cell Membranes

The signaling processes in our body occur in the cell membranes, but when they are damaged, they're prevented from receiving important messages from the brain and acting upon them. For example, the muscle cells may not respond properly to the messages from magnesium for relaxing, or insulin not being able to signal the cells to absorb more sugar.

Cause Hormonal Imbalance

Toxins have the ability to block, inhibit, and mimic hormones. For example, arsenic interferes with the thyroid receptors on the receiving cells. As a result, the cells don't get the messages from the thyroid hormones, which makes them rev up your body's metabolism. The result? You suffer from inexplicable fatigue. Toxins may also cause unexplained shifts in menstrual cycles in women, or cause extremes in hormone response in teenagers going through puberty.

Impair Your Ability to Detoxify Naturally

When your body is overwhelmed by a heavy toxic load, it becomes much harder for your system to naturally detoxify itself. The more you burden your body with harmful waste, the harder it is to get rid of it.

Do We Need to Detox?

When we do it right, detoxification helps improve our gut health and gives us an energy boost as well.

Think of it like taking care of your car. If you feed your gasoline engine with diesel, what would happen? It would splutter, cough, and stop working. Now, think of all the refined and processed foods that you are feeding your body. If you're going to be able to function at your best, you eventually reach a point where you need to flush all of the junk out and feed your system with premium fuel.

Refined foods are those that contain few or none of the essential nutrients like vitamins, minerals, and fiber that they might have had originally before being processed. Most of the time, these foods have more calories in comparison to their nutrients, and this mostly applies to those that are rich in carbohydrates, such as sugars and grains. When you replace these refined foods with whole, beneficial foods, such as fruits, vegetables, lean animal proteins, and whole grains, the stress in your digestive system eases. It also helps to repair damage in your body.

When you undertake a detox diet, you actually flush out your pipes. You move from a sluggish engine to enhanced acceleration and improved engine performance, which means you experience more energy.

Detox Myths Busted

Of course, detoxing your body seems like an amazing idea. Who doesn't want to do things that would get rid of the harmful waste from their body?

But is our body actually full of toxins?

Let us bust some common detox myths.

Myth: Our Body Requires Assistance to Detox

Fact: Our body does not **need** any kind of detox program. It's perfectly designed to be able to detoxify itself.

The toxins in our body come in two different forms:

- Endotoxins: These are the byproducts our body makes, like urea, lactic acid, and feces.
- Exotoxins: These are the substances that enter our body from the outside. They consist of chemicals

from the pesticides on food, cleaning products, cosmetics, and pollutants from water or the air.

The liver is our own efficient detoxification machine. Part of its job is to deal with the waste from the regular things we ingest through breathing or eating.

The most vital thing detoxification does is to help our body flush out this waste by taking care of the liver. Detoxification puts us on a path to maintaining a healthy diet and lifestyle so our organs don't get overwhelmed.

The key to this healthy, balanced diet is moderation. If you don't pack your liver full of the heavy waste from fat, alcohol, and sugar, then it will be able to keep going and do its job well. As long as it's healthy, it will handle all the things it needs to perfectly.

Myth: Detox Can Restore Our Health

Fact: If you overindulge with alcohol or unhealthy food on a regular basis, it can lead to damaging your liver. No detox diet can repair this damage.

Sugary drinks and fried foods are extremely difficult for your liver to process, and when excessive amounts of them build up in your liver, they are converted to fat. Once this fat starts to develop in your liver, it stays there for good. Even when you lose fat by reducing your overall body weight, the fat in your liver doesn't leave. This is called non-alcoholic fatty liver disease.

You can prevent more fat from entering your liver by limiting alcohol and consuming a healthy diet.

While you can't remove fat from your liver, when you shift from an unhealthy diet to a healthy, plant-based diet full of whole grains, lean proteins, vegetables, and fruits, you decrease stress on the liver and your other natural detoxification organs. This leads to benefits including improved digestion, more energy, reduced inflammation, and boosting your immune system.

Myth: All Detoxing Programs are Safe

Fact: Detox diets can be dangerous if not done correctly or if used for too long.

Often, people opt for complete fasting, juice-only fasting, or water fasting as methods of detoxification. Some also choose strict diets that consist only of vegetables and fruits or consume supplements, herbs, teas, or use enemas. When you follow strict routines like these for too long, it can lead to deficiencies of vitamins and minerals, electrolyte imbalance, fatigue, diarrhea, and stomach problems.

These regimes might appear harmless in the beginning since they only consist of natural foods and products. However, there is no conclusive evidence that this level of extreme detox works or is even safe.

Also, it's worth keeping in mind that commercial herbal supplements and detox programs do not necessarily get reviewed for their effectiveness and safety by the Food and Drug Administration before they are sold. So, there's no external scrutiny proving that they're without risk.

Furthermore, some herbal remedies are even toxic for your liver. If you think your body is deficient in a particular substance, consult your doctor and figure out what you might need to address the deficiency.

Myth: The Weight Loss from a Detox Diet is Sustainable

Fact: Effective detox diets are short-term and are therefore not a long-term strategy for weight loss.

Yes, you will probably drop some pounds when you are on a detox diet, but this is generally due to the loss of retained fluids and lean muscle mass. It's not the unhealthy body fat that you lose.

Detox plans are not meant to be maintained for an extended period, and it can affect your health negatively if you try to do so. Therefore, the results you notice will be temporary unless they lead to a healthier lifestyle overall.

Detox diets certainly have an impact on your body, but weight loss is a side effect of detoxification, not the main goal. If you're considering a weight loss plan or a detox diet, be sure that you talk to your healthcare professional first.

How to Know if You Need a Detox

Putting it simply, you need to detox when your body is overwhelmed with the toxins inside. These toxins are present in everyone's body and affects each of us differently. But some common signs that your body is harboring excess negative waste include enduring fatigue, bad skin, bloating from water retention, and weight problems.

The human body can and does detoxify itself naturally, but when it's constantly exposed to toxins without any relief, this process is compromised or slowed. At that point, our bodies start struggling to cleanse our tissues and organs properly. When you consume a diet rich in dairy, meat, and fatty or processed foods, it can clog your system. Irrespective of the diet you choose, how little your exposure to toxins, or the state of your detox mechanisms, everyone can benefit from the occasional detox. Think of it as rebooting your system and giving it a fresh start.

Why do You Need a Detox?

The process of detoxification is a natural part of how our bodies work. Without detox you would be sick all the time from the toxins present in the things you eat, drink, breathe, and touch. The world around us is filled with chemicals and other substances that are unusable by our bodies — and that's before we even consider man-made pollutants.

Even in a clean environment, waste is an issue your natural systems have to deal with. Our bodies produce toxic chemicals as byproducts to standard processes. For example, ethyl alcohol is produced within the body as food is broken down. In some cases, this can be further converted to acetaldehyde, an even more toxic substance This is all part of the body's normal function. Because it creates toxins it also has to eliminate them.

Have you seen advertisements about the importance of vitamins C and E for combating free radicals around us? Well, these free radicals are just more normal byproducts from chemical breakdown, but they are extremely toxic. These free radicals contribute to aging and can even lead to cancer. So you see, the systems that remove them from the body are critically important.

The Role of Organs in Detoxification

Several byproducts that result from the body's metabolism are simply waste that either are not needed or can't be used. Our bodies can even be damaged by these products. There are several mechanisms in our bodies whose functions get rid of these substances. Chemicals in our environment also cause pollute our bodies, and they too need to be neutralized or eliminated.

We've talked about the organs that work to detoxify the body. Let's go into a little more detail.

Lungs

Lungs remove toxic gases and volatile chemicals from our bodies when we breathe out. A good example of this is acetaldehyde, which is produced when our liver breaks down alcohol. Acetaldehyde creates the smell that emanates from a person who has had too much to drink, and the gas is lethal if it does not get removed from your blood and out of your body through your lungs.

Skin

Several toxins are eliminated from the body through being excreted in our sweat. Most of us believe that if we stimulate sweat by engaging in intense exercise or applying heat, it will lead to getting rid of toxins easily. Unfortunately, there is not enough evidence supporting this theory to consider it to be true. Also, if you sweat too much, it can lead to water loss and dehydration, which is even more harmful than the toxins.

Gastrointestinal System

Some of the waste that enters our bodies when we eat and drink gets removed through feces. This specifically applies when it comes to food poisoning or other substances that need to be ejected immediately. The body defends itself through diarrhea and vomiting to get rid of the toxins immediately.

Cell Operations of the Liver

All substances that get absorbed in our digestive tract are spread through the body through the veins. They drain the gut and carry everything into the gastrointestinal system. You can think of your liver as a gatekeeper between the intestines and blood circulation.

The liver breaks down matter into smaller parts that can be easily excreted. It also helps to destroy drugs, like nicotine, alcohol, and prescription medicines, since these are not natural to your body. Some of these medicines even have an adverse effect on your liver and damage its cells. It's sort of a war between the liver and the medicines you consume. The liver functions to destroy these foreign additives, even when they're helping your body, and sometimes these chemicals harm the liver even if they are good for other parts of your system.

Cell Operations of the Kidneys

The liver is the first organ to receive blood from your stomach and intestines. However, the blood that leaves your liver goes to your heart and is pumped directly to your kidneys. Kidneys help to regulate the salt and water balance in your body, but they also play a crucial role in the body's detoxification process. They filter waste substances out of the blood to be excreted in urine.

Key Takeaways

Our body has the capacity to naturally filter out the toxins we consume or that our systems create. However, if we eat a poor diet it can prevent the liver and gut from working at their optimum. For that reason, it's important to pay attention to what we feed our bodies so that we are taking care of our vital organs.

These toxins and chemicals contribute to several health issues. However, they can be eliminated or suppressed when we follow a detox diet. Let's look at the ways in which the detoxification process can help to eliminate these harmful substances to enable us to lead healthier and happier lives.

3

Detoxing to Reduce Bloating

You wake up and go to put on your favorite pair of jeans and realize you're not able to button them up. You quickly realize that you're going to have your period soon, or you've been up half the night dealing with painful bloating caused by something you ate.

Yes, we all get troubled by gas from time to time, but we are still embarrassed to talk about it to our doctor. Whether it was that Chinese buffet you went to last night, or an ice cream sundae, there have been times when we've had just too much to eat and had to get some relief by loosening the belt a couple of notches. However, there are several things that can cause bloating, it's not just from food.

About 10-20 percent of adults complain of excessive flatulence or belching. But gas or bloating does not necessarily mean that there's something wrong with your digestion. However, if you wish to reduce gas and the embarrassment it causes, you first need to focus on your eating habits and diet.

What is Bloating?

Bloating can be the result of water retention, swelling, or gaseous pressure. Bloating feels different from one person to the other. However, it generally refers to the feeling of being full or larger than before around the lower abdomen. It can be very uncomfortable. If you're dealing with generalized bloating, it means that your entire body is holding on to more water than it should be. However, there is also localized bloating that occurs when one or more organs of your body are swollen and causing discomfort.

When you feel bloated, it can be quite tricky to determine the exact cause, since bloating is a term used to describe the overall feeling of tightness. Both swelling and bloating can lead to several problems, so it is best to know what you're dealing with.

Causes of Bloating

Overeating

When we think of bloating, we often connect it to a large meal like a Thanksgiving dinner. There's a good reason for that: one of the most common causes of bloating is overeating. To control your portion sizes, especially at a large family party that is focused around food, you can try using a smaller plate. This will help you eat comparatively less in one sitting. Also, slow down while you eat to give your body time to digest the food. It typically takes several minutes for the signals of fullness from the stomach to reach the brain. When you eat too quickly, you are often over-full and uncomfortable by the time your stomach tells your brain you need to stop eating.

Food Intolerance

Generally, when you feel bloated, it's due to excessive intake of food or fluid. But when you have not eaten much and still feel like your belly is tight and distended, it might be because you have eaten something that has disagreed with you. Certain food sensitivities or intolerances, such as gluten, dairy, and acidic or spicy foods, can lead to your gastrointestinal tract facing a more difficult time than usual.

When these food intolerances remain undiagnosed and you eat items that your body can't deal with, it leads to bloating. Your normal systems try to break down the food, but it results in a lot of gas.

If you have this experience frequently, try to keep a food journal. You can track everything you consume, how often you observe bloating, and the kind of discomfort you face. That way you can identify exactly what specific foods are triggering your problems.

High-Sodium or High-Starch Food

Foods that contain a lot of salt can cause water retention and eating starchy foods can lead to increased amounts of gaseous bloating.

Processed Food

Packaged foods are definitely convenient for snacking and when you need a quick meal. However, this food is usually processed and is not only high in sodium, but often also contains chemicals, including monosodium glutamate (MSG). This ingredient makes you feel like you had the entire day's meals in one go. MSG is commonly found in packaged meals, Chinese food, and in sauces and dressings on buffets.

Eating Too Late

According to an old myth, if you eat close to your bedtime, you will gain weight. However, this is not necessarily true. You actually gain weight when you consume more calories than you burn. But when you have a heavy meal before you go to bed, you can feel as though you've gained weight overnight.

When you're sleeping, your body is busy repairing tissue and performing daily housekeeping on your organs. The brain, heart and other muscles completely relax, and that means there's less focus on the digestive system. For that reason, you don't digest your food as well while sleeping as when you're awake. Furthermore, food digests more slowly when you're in a reclined position. This all adds up to discomfort in the night that continues into the morning, when you usually feel refreshed and at your leanest.

Drinking Soda

Carbonated beverages, like soda and sparkling water, can result in bloating. The fizz in your soda — even in the diet ones — can be trapped in your stomach. This eventually leads to belching and bloating.

You can avoid this problem by limiting your consumption of soda and switching to a healthier option. Consume water with cucumber or lemon with your meals. If you need that caffeine kick early in the afternoon, drink green tea. If you feel bloated already, try having peppermint tea. It's one of the most common remedies to reduce the discomfort caused by bloating.

Swallowing Air

You will also feel over-full when you swallow a lot of air. This usually happens when you are chewing gum, drinking through a straw, or eating too fast. Sometimes belching will ease this type of bloating.

Undiagnosed Health Conditions

There are certain health conditions that cause swelling or bloating. Liver and heart diseases and venous insufficiency all make excess fluid gather in your limbs or abdomen. These conditions have prominent symptoms which should be examined by your healthcare provider for proper identification.

Certain chronic conditions can lead to distension in specific areas. If you have a family history of this type of condition, or a specific concern, you should consult with your doctor to rule them out.

There are also many gastrointestinal conditions that can lead to stomach ailments and bloating, such as irritable bowel syndrome, Crohn's disease, and ulcerative colitis. Acid reflux and medications to treat it can also result in an uncomfortable increase of gas in your abdomen.

Certain Medications

Apart from the drugs to relieve acid reflux, there are several other medications that cause bloating. Medicines to soften stools can make you feel gassy. There are also several birth control hormones, in the form of either pills, implants, or patches that can make a woman feel heavy and swollen.

Other medicines for diarrhea, narcotic pain relievers, aspirin, and iron or fiber supplements can lead to several gastrointestinal symptoms. If you feel your medicines are the cause of your bloating, talk to your doctor. But in the meantime, don't stop taking prescribed medication without consulting your physician.

Of course, every person is different, and what causes bloating in one will not necessarily have the same impact on another. It's all about learning what food gives you discomfort and limiting its quantity in your diet.

There are specific over-the-counter medicines, like antacids, that can be used for relief from discomfort caused by food. These drugs enable the gaseous buildup to pass more freely through your body and reduce bloating. But you must keep in mind that not all over-the-counter medications work in the same fashion. Talk to your doctor or pharmacist and inform them about your symptoms so they can help you choose the right kind of medication for your problem.

The Passing of Gas Through the Body

The three common ways by which we expel gas from our bodies are through abdominal bloating, burping, and flatus. The air we swallow, which can stay in our stomach for some time, gets released by belching. Bloating generally occurs when air gets trapped in the colon or small bowel and can't be released. The air that passes through the bowel is generally in the form of flatus which is normally emitted about 12-15 times a day. The gas in the intestines increases as the day goes along.

This gas contains carbon dioxide, nitrogen, methane, and hydrogen, and can result from several different factors, including your eating behavior and bacterial fermentation of foods.

Bacterial Fermentation

The colon is filled with yeast, fungi, and bacteria that break down the foods that are not digested by our small intestine. By this point in the digestive system, these foods are typically just different forms of carbohydrates. The bacteria consume these undigested carbohydrates, and the resulting fermentation leads to the production of methane and hydrogen gases being expelled from the body as flatus. One of the most common sources of carbohydrates that cause gas is lactose — a sugar found in dairy products. People who are lactose intolerant lack the enzyme lactase, which is required to digest this form of carbohydrate. The second most common carbohydrate that leads to gas is beans. They contain indigestible raffinose that leads to flatus.

Behaviors, Activity, Food Choices

Your eating behavior and other habits including gulping foods, chewing gum, and drinking while eating can make you swallow a lot of air. Bulky foods like cabbage, lettuce, and dense pieces of bread when not chewed properly into smaller pieces can also increase the amount of air swallowed.

Generally, the air that is swallowed consists of carbon dioxide, nitrogen, and oxygen. It does not have a foul smell but plays a role in creating gas and discomfort.

Different people are sensitive in different ways when it comes to gas production. Consider keeping a food journal to determine if your gas is related to specific foods or behaviors.

Food Choices and Behavior that Lead to Gas

Foods

- Fried, fatty, or spicy foods
- Carbonated drinks
- Dried fruits
- Cabbage, onions, broccoli
- Legumes
- Prune or apple juice
- Anything that contains mannitol, maltitol, or sorbitol, ingredients typically found in sugar-free or low-carb foods

Behaviors

- Eating when you're upset
- Overloading your stomach with food
- Sighing while you eat
- Chewing tobacco or smoking
- Drinking extremely hot or cold beverages

- Drinking from a straw or a sports bottle
- Drinking from a water fountain
- Wearing tightly fitting outfits
- Consuming cold-relief medicines over a long time
- Eating hard candies or chewing gum

How to Choose the Best Non-Gassy Foods

Why Some Foods Cause Gas

Gassy foods are those that contain the specific carbohydrates that come from sugar or starch or soluble fiber from most fruits and certain vegetables like beans and peas. The small intestine has limited or none of the enzymes needed to digest these substances, so they pass directly through to the large intestine where there are more gut bacteria to break down the food. These bacteria produce gas that contains sulfur, which is what causes flatulence to sometimes smell bad.

If you want to avoid gas, there are some foods that are less likely to create it. By choosing foods that are lower in carbohydrates, you enable them to be broken down before reaching the large intestine. They are therefore less likely to cause you embarrassment in public.

Animal Proteins

Our body is designed to efficiently digest proteins. The protein that comes from animal sources don't contain carbohydrates, so there is nothing in them to feed the gut bacteria. This makes protein ideal food when you're trying to avoid gas or bloating.

Gravies, sauces and glazes often contain added onions, garlic, and sugars. These can all lead to gas, so for the best result, eat your protein sources without anything added:

- Eggs
- Chicken
- Beef
- Turkey
- Fish

If you don't eat animal products, there are also plenty of vegetarian and vegan options to choose.

Vegetables

There are many vegetables that have lower carbohydrate content and so don't contribute to the intestinal fermentation that causes gas.

These vegetables are all good for you, even if you're trying to avoid bloat, so it's safe to pile them up on your plate.

- Cucumber
- Bell peppers
- Fennel
- Bok choy
- Lettuce
- Tomatoes
- Spinach
- Zucchini
- Green beans
- Greens like spinach or kale

Fruits

Certain fruits are known to produce less gas than some other forms of carbohydrate. However, it's a good idea to eat them in moderation. The following are considered to be those least likely to cause a build up of gas.

- Grapes
- Strawberries
- Raspberries
- Pineapple
- Blueberries
- Kiwi
- Cantaloupe
- Honeydew
- Clementine

Fermented Foods

The bacteria that are found naturally in fermented foods already take care of the carbohydrates that your gut would otherwise need to deal with. This relieves your intestine from doing the hard work, which reduces the chances of creating gas.

An added benefit of these natural bacteria is that they also help to maintain the overall health of your gut. As long as you have no allergy or intolerance, you can't go wrong with these choices.

- Yogurt without added sugars
- Kombucha
- Fermented vegetables

- Kefir

Grains

You might be surprised to know that there are specific carbohydrates in wheat and wheat products that lead to gas. In order to avoid gas and flatulence, you can substitute the following options for wheat-based items.

- Rice bread
- Gluten-free bread
- Quinoa
- Oats
- White or brown rice

Snacks

Apart from the non-gassy fruits and veggies, there are other great snack options that you can grab when you need a quick bite. These include nuts, however, not all nuts are reliably low-gas, so it's best to limit yourself to walnuts, macadamias, and pecans.

It's important to note that most of the items on our list of foods that can cause gas are actually good for us. The fiber and iron content in legumes, for example, are easily digested and perform an important job by helping to move material through the digestive system. When you eat these foods more regularly your body becomes accustomed to the starches and the gas production will decrease.

How to Beat Bloating: Detox Drinks for a Flatter Belly

First, let's understand that bloating is a natural part of our lives. When your intestines are doing their jobs, you will experience some extra gas. Or you may just be a bit puffy from the salt on your french fries. Whatever the reason for your discomfort from bloat, these detox drinks can provide some relief.

De-Bloat Detox Drink

Need more lemon and green tea in your diet? Who doesn't! These ingredients will rev up your digestive system. Since most bloating is a result of the activities of your intestines, it's relieved faster when you move things along a bit.

Simply boil a cup of water, add green tea and the juice of half a lemon, plus a handful of fresh mint leaves. Voilà! An effective de-bloating detox drink that's ready in no time.

Detox Cucumber Lemonade

Vitamin C helps to keep your immune system in top form, and this lemonade will also help to sooth inflammation.

To make this detox lemonade, blend and strain one chopped cucumber. Mix it with water warm enough to melt a little honey, top it up with ice and freshly squeezed lemon juice. You will feel more refreshed, hydrated, and less swollen too, if the bloating you're experiencing is due to inflammation.

Coconut Water Electrolyte Drink

Did you know that constipation can also lead to an uncomfortable, distended abdomen?

You can both improve your hydration and get your digestive system going to relieve these conditions. Electrolytes are crucial when it comes to hydrating your body, and coconut water helps your body to absorb them.

To make this electrolyte drink, steep about 4 ounces of hot green tea. Mix in 8 ounces of coconut water and the juice of a lemon. Add in a few ice cubes and sip until it's finished.

How to Detox and Reduce Bloating

Let us discuss the ways in which you can detox and reduce bloating.

Drink Only Tea or Water

When people are bloated, they often skip drinking water as they feel it would worsen their situation. However, the opposite is actually true because your body holds on to fluids through water retention in an effort to prevent dehydration. So if you make sure to consume plenty of water, it signals to your body that it doesn't need to retain any of it in order to stay hydrated. Fluids — and especially water — are absolutely essential for proper digestion.

Have A Banana

Bananas are rich in potassium, a nutrient that works to regulate the fluid balance in your body and flatten your belly bloat. Potassium can also offset the effects of excess sodium in your diet, which is one of the primary causes of water retention.

Avoid Specific Vegetables

Although they are packed with health-promoting nutrients, foods that are rich in FODMAPs (or fermentable carbohydrates) can be sneaky belly-bloaters as well. The reason is poor absorption of sugars and carbohydrates or a lack of sufficient water. To stave off bloating, limit your consumption of the following vegetables.

- Cabbage
- White onions
- Broccoli
- Cauliflower
- Artichokes
- Brussels sprouts

Don't Chew Gum

When you chew gum, it not only enables the tummy-bloating air to enter your body, but it may also contain artificial sweeteners and sugar alcohols such as xylitol and sorbitol. Since these sugar alcohols cannot be absorbed by your body, they can result in bloating and discomfort.

Have Dinner Early

Intermittent fasting has become very popular in recent years because of its science-backed benefits for weight loss. However, for most of us, not consuming food for 16 hours a day might sound unrealistic. But let me tell you a secret — you fast each night when you're asleep, which is why the first meal of the day is called "breakfast" — you're breaking the fast. And that period of sleep can form part of your fasting window each day.

The longer this period of fasting is stretched out, the fewer calories you consume. And the fewer calories you take in, the less chance there is that you will eat something that will disagree your digestion. Try to cut off your food intake by 7 p.m., or by 8 p.m. at the latest. You can also delay your breakfast. That way, the fasting period doesn't sound so difficult, does it? Be sure to keep a gap of at least 12 hours between your last meal at night and your first meal the next day. This gives your digestive system enough time to recover, and you'll notice your belly bloat disappearing faster than ever.

We'll talk more about fasting, and intermittent fasting in particular, in a later chapter.

Consume a High-Protein Breakfast

Once your digestive system is awake, start your day by consuming protein. We all get busy with our daily schedules throughout the day, but when we consume a high-protein breakfast, it can prevent energy crashes later. These dips often lead us to reach for caffeinated beverages or processed foods that have a higher ratio of bloat-inducing constituents, such as sodium.

Have Ginger Tea

When your digestive system is sluggish, your metabolism rate slows down simultaneously. You can wake up your system by starting your day with a cup of ginger tea. This drink is not only fasting-friendly, but it will also help to improve your digestion and bowel movements. Don't like ginger? Try mixing it with lemon or lime. You can also try out other kinds of teas that work as effective remedies for bloat, like peppermint, chamomile or fennel.

Have Multiple Small Meals

To keep your metabolism going throughout the day, consider eating small fiber and protein-packed meals or snacks every three to four hours. You will not just burn more calories but eating more frequently will also prevent those afternoon crashes and slumps at the end of the day.

Until you get used to the routine, it can be hard to fit so many small meals into a day. Try using your phone to set reminders for these intervals. Here are some ideas for healthy snacks:

- A handful of berries and nuts
- Apple and peanut butter
- Vegetables and hummus
- Yogurt and granola

Eat Slowly to Prevent Gulping Air

It's understandable that when you're back home after a long, tiring day, you are famished and ready to eat whatever is available, and fast. But eating too quickly makes you swallow excess air, which leads to that bloating and gas you're trying to avoid. When you slow down the chewing process with your mouth closed, it has the opposite effect. You might find it useful to snack on a piece of fruit or a handful of nuts before your dinner is ready in order to resist the temptation to gobble down your meal.

Skip Your Morning Coffee

As much as we all love having our morning coffee, consuming it when you're trying to combat belly bloat is a no-no, unfortunately.

Consuming drinks that are high in caffeine or sugar not only dehydrates your body, but it often adds to your calorie intake as well. If your body is dehydrated, it will hold on to any of the water it has, and this causes that bloated feeling. Try a glass of water with lemon juice instead to brighten up your morning.

Avoid Eating Beans

Several types of beans, including soybeans, contain oligosaccharides. These are non-digestible molecules of sugar that our bodies cannot break down completely, which leads to bloating and gas. While it may be easy to avoid including beans in your meals, if you look, you'll find that they come from some surprising sources. You probably wouldn't think of beans when you're unwrapping your favorite protein bar, but many of them actually contain protein derived from soybeans. So, it pays to check your labels.

Consume More Fiber and Avoid Refined Flour

Foods that are made from white flour, such as white bread, white rice, and white pasta, are low in fiber and can cause you to get a little backed up. Instead, try swapping out these white carbs for their whole-grain alternatives. Making a simple switch from white bread to whole grain bread or white rice to brown rice will give your diet a fiber boost and ease any tendency you have to constipation.

The following high-fiber foods don't contain any indigestible fibers.

- Whole-grain bread
- Brown rice
- Carrots
- Nuts
- Chia and flax seeds
- Berries like raspberries and blackberries
- Acorn squash

Avoid Greasy Foods

Foods that are loaded with fats, such as deep-fried food and most takeout meals, lead to an upset gastrointestinal tract. Of course, there are some fats that are great for gut health, such as the omega-3s found in oily fish or nuts. However, greasy food doesn't interact with your body in the same fashion. Fast food typically contains a high level of unhealthy fat, such as trans fat and saturated fat. In addition to loading you up with a lot of surplus calories, all this fat causes an inflammatory response in your body. That means that your system has to work extra-hard to get it all out.

Limit Alcohol

Alcohol damages your digestive tract directly and causes a series of reactions that negatively affect your health. First of all, it destroys a lot of the good gut bacteria, which is bad for your overall well-being. What's more, when you specifically try to get rid of bloating, alcohol inhibits your digestion process and leads to dehydration. This makes your digestive tract slow down, resulting in constipation.

When you consume alcohol, your body switches to working on removing the alcohol and not digesting food. This causes a bloated tummy.

Avoiding alcoholic drinks is one of the cornerstones of a successful detox.

Cut Down on Dairy

As we age, dairy products can be problematic for our stomachs since many adults produce less lactase, the digestive enzyme that digests lactose. If you eat dairy products regularly and are having abdominal pain or bloating, try cutting dairy from your diet for a couple of days and see how your body reacts to it. Some items, like cheese and yogurt with live enzymes, may be less troublesome than pasteurized products such as milk and ice cream.

Avoid Sweeteners - Both Real and Artificial

Food that contains processed sugar — especially artificial sweeteners — are particularly upsetting to your digestive tract and lead to gas and bloating. Also, artificial sweeteners like sugar alcohols are constituents of poorly digested FODMAPs that will only increase your problems.

Consume Smaller Portions

Eating a large meal will leave you feeling inflated, and this is not what you're looking for at the end of your detox period when you have just managed to debloat. Eat your food slowly and put your spoon or fork down between every bite. A good guide to portion control is to eat until you're about 90 percent full and then stop. This gives time for your brain to decide if you're really still hungry. You can also practice portion control by measuring out all your meals before you eat.

Limit High-Sodium Foods

While they might taste great, high-sodium food items are bad for your stomach and intestine and when you eat them will result in temporary weight gain and water retention. If you overload your system with salt, your kidneys struggle to keep up. In addition to causing bloating, it can contribute to serious conditions like kidney disease, kidney stones, and high blood pressure. If you want to get rid of bloating, you should first assess the amount of sodium you are consuming each day.

Cut back on sodium-rich foods by following these tips:

- Swap canned foods for fresh or frozen foods
- Look for canned foods with lower or no salt
- Avoid processed meats and replace them with baked or grilled lean protein
- Use different spices to season your food instead of simply relying on salt.
- If you consume a lot of fast food, seek out low-sodium options
- Avoid soda and other drinks with high sodium content.

Avoid Carbonated Beverages

While you're sipping on your favorite carbonated drink, it's most likely contributing to your swollen feeling with each mouthful. This is because the bubbles temporarily inflate your stomach. Diet soda is the worst culprit for this since, in addition to the bubbles, the artificial sweeteners will leave you feeling worse than before.

Choose Diuretic, Electrolyte-Rich Foods

Foods like honeydew melon, cranberries, and celery have diuretic properties that help to fight water retention. In fact, honeydew is rich in potassium to help displace sodium and flush out the excess water from your body. It acts as a natural replacement for electrolytes, making it one of the best foods to combat bloating!

Key Takeaways

Bloating is caused by a combination of food choices and behaviors that affect the gut. However, a good detox is all your body needs to improve digestion and reduce bloating.

Some food and lifestyle choices affect the amount and types of bacteria present in our gut. Upsetting this balance will contribute to bloating and other digestive problems. In addition, an overabundance of unhelpful bacteria will encourage inflammation in the gut.

Let's look at how detoxing helps us deal with gut inflammation.

4

Detoxing Can Reduce Gut Inflammation

D id you know that your body contains 10 times more bacteria than cells? In most people, the immune system protects your body against bacterial invaders without causing constant inflammation. But by understanding how this process works, you can determine what to do when it doesn't work. This can help treat inflammatory bowel conditions like ulcerative colitis and Crohn's disease.

Just like any other organ in our bodies, the gastrointestinal tract can be affected by chronic inflammation. The constant activation of the immune system that occurs in our joints, leading to inflammatory arthritis, and in our arteries, leading to plaque buildup, can also happen in our gastrointestinal tract. It damages the lining of the intestine and several other parts of the digestive system. Gut inflammation is the cause of conditions like celiac disease or inflammatory bowel disease (IBD).

Healthy Gut Bacteria

Gut bacteria are one of the most influential yet overlooked bacteria in our body. But they are now associated with several health issues and solutions.

There are many things you can do to maintain the health of your gut bacteria. Let's look at what your gut flora is, what can disturb its balance, and what you can do to help it thrive.

What is Gut Flora?

The human gut flora is also called microflora, microbiome, or microbiota. They make up a world of microorganisms that flourish in our gastrointestinal tract and help us to properly digest the foods and liquids that we consume. It's estimated that there is about 100 trillion of this gut flora, known as microbes. It typically consists of various strains of bacteria, but there are also some kinds of fungi and protozoa.

This proliferation of gut flora is essential to our health, but it's interesting that we are not born with it. We get our gut flora from our mother when we are born.

A significant difference has been found between the flora of a breast-fed infant and one that is formula fed. When a breast-fed infant is weaned, their flora has a close resemblance to that of their mother. A formula-fed infant will have a narrower band of flora and may have more stomach problems early in life until their gut flora fully develops.

The relationship we have with our gut bacteria is usually mutually beneficial. Our gut flora contributes to our good health in several ways.

- Keeps harmful bacteria at bay
- Promotes digestion
- Stimulates the immune system
- Supports gut motility
- Synthesizes vitamins
- Helps absorb nutrients

What Can Hurt Gut Bacteria

When our health is optimal, good gut bacteria help to keep the potentially problematic bacteria in check. When this balance is disrupted, it's known as dysbiosis and can lead to a range of health challenges.

There are several factors that have a negative impact on the health of gut flora, which includes:

- Modern diet
- Physical stress
- Psychological health
- Antibiotic use
- Radiation
- Peristalsis dysfunction

When Gut Bacteria Goes Bad

Intestinal dysbiosis is related to several chronic illnesses that include:

- Irritable bowel syndrome (IBS)
- Inflammatory bowel disease (IBD) including ulcerative colitis and Crohn's disease
- Atopic dermatitis or eczema, which is an inflammatory skin condition
- Ankylosing spondylitis, which refers to a type of inflammatory arthritis affecting your spine

Signs Your Gut is Unhealthy

Several factors that characterize our modern day-to-day lives can damage our gut flora. Our tendency to consume high-sugar and processed foods and get too little sleep, our high stress levels, and even the antibiotics we take to cure infections all negatively affect the bacteria that live in our guts. This disruption, in turn, affects other aspects of our health, including our immune system, heart, brain, hormone levels, weight, skin, our body's ability to absorb nutrients, and can even play a role in the development of cancer.

There are several ways in which the unhealthy gut manifests itself.

Upset Stomach

If your stomach is feeling out of sorts with symptoms like bloating, constipation, gas, heartburn, or diarrhea, you may have an unhealthy gut. When your gut is unbalanced, it is more difficult for you to process and digest your food and eliminate waste.

A High-Sugar Diet

If you are consuming a lot of processed food and sugar, it can destroy good bacteria in your gut. This creates an imbalance that increases sugar cravings, which can then lead to even more damage to your gut. Processed sugars — typically high-fructose corn syrup —are linked to increased inflammation in your body.

Unintentional Changes in Weight

When you gain or lose weight without making any significant changes in your exercise or diet habits, it's a sign that your gut is not healthy. When you have an imbalanced gut, your body's ability to absorb nutrients, store fat, and regulate blood sugar levels are all impaired. Losing weight is a result of small intestinal bacterial growth (SIBO), while gaining weight is a sign that you are developing resistance to insulin or you have the urge to overeat because of poor absorption of nutrients.

Sleep Disturbance and Constant Fatigue

An unhealthy gut creates disturbances in your sleeping patterns which, over time, will cause chronic fatigue. The majority of your body's serotonin, a hormone that affects your sleep and mood, gets produced in your gut. This serotonin production can be slowed or halted when the gut is damaged or working poorly.

Skin Irritation

A skin condition called eczema is related to poor gut health. Inflammation in your gut caused by food allergies or poor diet can lead to increased leaking of specific proteins into your body. These proteins cause the skin to be dry, itchy and to develop sores, a condition that has to be treated both on the outside and the inside.

Autoimmune Conditions

It's known that an unhealthy gut is connected to an increase in systemic inflammation and alteration of the proper functioning of your immune system. This causes autoimmune diseases, which cause your body to attack its own cells instead of the harmful invaders.

Food Intolerances

Several food sensitivities are caused by digestive malfunction. However, this is different from being allergic to a particular food item, which happens due to a reaction of your immune system. Food intolerances are related to an unhealthy gut and poor quality of beneficial gut bacteria. This leads to difficulty in digesting the trigger foods, and the resultant unpleasant side effects of gas, diarrhea, bloating, nausea, and abdominal pain.

How Gut Flora Impacts Health

Development

Babies are born with either completely or mostly sterile intestines. During birth they are exposed to the microorganisms in their mother's birth canal, and this is where the microbiome population originates. The microbiome is further populated through environmental exposure and consuming breast milk, formula milk, and eventually food.

Location

The substances that are secreted during the digestion process have a direct impact on where the gut bacteria proliferate. Bile, stomach acid, and several pancreatic enzymes prevent bacterial colonization in your stomach or in the first parts of your small intestine.

Gut bacteria are found in smaller quantities in the last portions of your small intestine; however, they are found mainly in the large intestine. This entire world of microbiomes is separated from the rest of your body internally via a single layer of cells present in your large intestine, known as epithelial tissue.

Functions

As we've seen, your gut flora plays a critical role in maintaining your overall health. Their most essential functions are protecting your immune system and enhancing your body's metabolism.

Supporting the Immune System

There are two main ways in which our gut bacteria support our immune system. The first way is that the helpful gut flora offers direct protection to the lining of our intestines, known as the epithelial cells. These cells keep substances that are harmful to us at bay and contained within the intestine where they can be flushed away. When this system is compromised, increased intestinal permeability develops, a condition known as leaky gut syndrome.

The second way is that the favorable bacteria in our guts work with our immune system to fight disease. This is at the level of the lining of our intestines, which helps to fight against several disease-causing bacteria and other harmful substances.

Helpful Metabolic Effects

The gut bacteria in our body ensure we absorb all the essential nutrients such as vitamins, minerals, etc. They also deal with the carbohydrates that don't get digested in the small intestine. This interaction provides us with more nutrients, modulates the storage of fat, and encourages the growth of epithelial cells.

Other Associated Health Problems

We know now that when there is an imbalance of gut bacteria in the body, it can lead to several health problems, both digestive and non-digestive. Health issues that are directly linked to the disruption of gut flora, include the following:

- Diabetes
- Inflammatory bowel disease (IBD)
- Inflammatory bowel syndrome (IBS)
- Atopic diseases
- Metabolic syndrome
- Obesity

How to Care for Your Gut Flora

When you keep your stress levels low, consume a well-balanced diet full of nutrients, and minimize the consumption of antibiotics, you can enhance the health of your gut flora.

Gut Bacteria and Detox

When you incorporate certain dietary changes in your routine, it helps keep your gut bacteria happy.

Decrease Refined Carbohydrates

Refined carbohydrates, including sugar, are foods that interact with your gut bacteria through the process of fermentation and contribute to excess bloating and gas. Decreasing or eliminating such food from your diet eases the digestive system.

Get to Know Your Prebiotics

As you learn more and more about your gut bacteria, you will also learn about prebiotics. These are the ingredients found in food items that encourage the growth of healthy gut bacteria. They are typically found in fruits and vegetables that contain higher amounts of soluble and insoluble fiber.

If you have heard of the buzzwords "inulin" and "fructooligosaccharides" (FOS), then you might know that these refer to prebiotic components and that they are extremely beneficial to your gut flora. The following foods are all good sources of FOS.

- Bananas
- Artichokes
- Rye
- Chicory
- Garlic
- Blueberries
- Leeks
- Asparagus
- Onions

Consume More Fermented Foods

Fermented foods are the ones that contain live cultures of beneficial bacterial strains. This sounds exotic, but when you take a look at the list of foods included, you might already be familiar with a few of them.

- Kombucha
- Kimchi
- Kefir
- Sauerkraut - not the canned one, but the raw and unpasteurized one that you find in the refrigerators of your grocery store
- Live yogurt

Add Bone Broth to Your Diet

Several health practitioners have suggested that eating bone broth is healthy and healing for your gut. While the evidence is inconclusive, such broths contain an abundance of vitamins, minerals, and natural gelatins. They are also good for hydration and balancing electrolytes.

Lifestyle Changes for Healthy Gut Bacteria

As you have seen, one of the biggest challenges to keeping your insides healthy is taking care of your gut bacteria. When the gut microbiome is in balance, then digestion is enabled and absorption of the vital nutrients and minerals your body needs works better. Here are some things you can do in your daily lifestyle to optimize your inner health.

Minimal Antibiotic Usage

With all the wonderful advances in medical science it's often tempting to demand that every small ailment should have an easy solution. It's common for people to want antibiotics for every ailment, but the truth is that antibiotics don't work in all cases. What's more, they destroy not only the harmful bacteria in your body, but also the good. When you're unwell work with your doctor to determine the cause of the illness and the best possible resolution. Whenever possible, avoid antibiotics for viral or mild illness.

Stress Management Skills

Human life is filled with stressors which can cause damage to our gut bacteria when we make unhealthy eating choices or suffer increased inflammation and illness as a side effect of anxiety. As you learn and apply skills to control your stress you will decrease the wear and tear on your body, down to the microscopic level. When stress is high, remember to be mindful of the little things you can do that can have a big impact, such as deep breathing, exercise, stretching, meditation, and maintaining a healthy diet.

Key Takeaways

Gut inflammation is caused by the poor condition of or damage to your gut bacteria or as a symptom of chronic disease. It leads to health problems ranging from chronic constipation to fatigue and irregular periods.

However, a detox diet along with good lifestyle changes are key to improving your gut health and controlling these symptoms. When you make even a few small changes, it helps to strengthen the gut flora, which, in turn, assists the reduction of gut inflammation and better digestion.

5

Detoxing Can Clear Your Foggy Brain

D id you know that when your body is not working at its best, it directly impacts the functioning of your brain?

If you have ever felt fuzzy-headed or unable to focus, what you're dealing with is brain fog. It is not a medical condition or a formal diagnosis, but it's a real phenomenon. Brain fog refers to difficulties with memory, logic, focus, and problem-solving. It can be a sign of an underlying health condition that needs a doctor's attention, but often it's related to your diet and overall health, both things that can be improved with detoxing and healthy lifestyle changes.

Brain fog can be the result of several factors, but all of them make you feel like you're out of sorts or not your normal self. It can even leave you feeling a bit crazy and affect your ability to work as well as your day-to-day life and relationships.

What is Brain Fog?

Brain fog is usually a symptom rather than a condition or a diagnosis. It usually presents as having difficulty thinking clearly or remembering basic things. Some people describe is as feeling like their head is stuffed with cotton candy.

When you're suffering from brain fog, you might not be able to concentrate on work for very long. It might be difficult to focus on conversations or even these words that you're reading. Making up your mind or making decisions, irrespective of them being small or big, can even be challenging. You may find you need more and more coffee or other stimulants to help you focus, and it can be tempting to eat more to try to stay awake. In more severe cases, you might also experience headaches, difficulty with your vision, and even nausea.

What Causes Brain Fog?

Brain fog is a symptom associated with sleep disorders, depression, nutrient deficiency, over-consumption of sugar or stimulants, a thyroid condition, or menopause. Other common causes include either eating too much and frequently, not getting proper sleep, inactivity, poor diet, and chronic stress. Let's look at a few of these situations in more depth.

Hormonal Changes

Everyone — both men and women — experiences changes in hormones throughout their lives. These may be tied to big physical changes such as pregnancy, menopause, puberty, and decreasing testosterone and estrogen due to aging. They may also be related to changes in your lifestyle and environment, including changing sleep patterns and diet. When your hormones are changing or unstable it affects your ability to think clearly as your body tries to regulate itself.

Disturbed Sleep

Poor sleeping habits include irregular sleeping and waking times, sleeping for less than seven to eight hours, or exposure to blue light before you go to bed. Problems with sleep can disturb the natural circadian rhythm in your body, which is your body's internal clock. This often leads to brain fog. Studies surrounding blue light exposure, such as the light emitted by computers and smartphones, show that the blue wavelengths in the light decrease melatonin, a hormone that is vital for deep REM sleep.

Both REM and non-REM sleep are needed to process memories from your day and enable you to heal from the day's exertions and experiences. The hours from 10 pm to 2 am are those in which your body and brain naturally detoxify the most. Hence, when you remain active during these hours or if you can't get into deep enough sleep, your body's natural detoxification process is disrupted and can lead to fogginess.

On the other hand, having an untimely wake up that interrupts your sleep cycle also leads to impairing the cognitive functions of your brain. This can apply to sleeping too much as well as too little. When your deep sleep is disturbed, you don't breathe as deeply, so your body isn't getting the amount of oxygen it needs. What's more, too much sleep may interrupt the eating schedule that's good for your body. You might miss medications or other important cues for your brain. You may have heard someone complain that they feel worse after oversleeping than they did before they went to bed. This is a real issue, and it also contributes to brain fog.

Remember that if you hit the snooze button on your alarm, it won't actually help you get enough rest. Instead, it increases the chance that you'll fall back asleep only to be disrupted again. Most of the time you will feel better if you just get up and get going.

Food Sensitivities and Diet Deficiencies

We've discussed how your brain and your gut are connected, so it should come as little surprise that food intolerances and diet deficiencies cause brain fog. Studies show, for example, that the consumption of gluten by someone who has an intolerance for it results in cognitive dysfunction related to an increased inflammatory response. Simply put, your body is too busy fighting the intolerance to think clearly!

So you can see that it's important to identify and address food intolerances. You can identify them by working with a doctor or nutritionist or by eliminating certain foods —like gluten — from your diet and monitoring the changes in your health. Depending on the outcome of your experiment, you should then consider very slowly reintroducing them again, one at a time, and monitor the effect on your body and brain. Often our bodies just need a break and then when the foods are reintroduced, we are much better able to tolerate them. Obviously with allergies or severe intolerances, talk to your doctor first before embarking on this plan.

In our fast moving, highly processed way of life, few people get all the vitamins and nutrients they need, and these vitamins are important. For example, vitamin B12 helps form the red blood cells in your body and maintains the central nervous system. Vitamin C helps bolster the immune system. Vitamin D assists in protecting the bones, immunity, and mood control. Vitamins and minerals are essential to maintaining our physical and psychological systems, and most of us don't get all of the vitamins we need from the food we consume. Again, this is associated with fuzzy thinking and being over-tired. A healthy, balanced diet — sometimes with the addition of a daily multi-vitamin — can help give our bodies these building blocks that are so important for good health and a clear mind.

Stress

Stress is often treated as a common and harmless term to describe the lives most of us live. It's even purported that you need a little stress in order to be motivated and success-ful. While it's true that a little stress drives us to work harder, when you suffer from chronic stress, it can create havoc on your body.

When you experience a stressful situation, your body's fight-or-flight response is activated by the sympathetic nervous system, or SNS. This response releases norepinephrine and epinephrine, also known as adrenaline. The release of these hormones diverts your body's energy away from its usual functions to focus on the stressors. This can make it difficult for you to concentrate or think clearly and leads to your brain becoming exhausted and foggy.

If removing the stressful situations from your life isn't an option, you can learn to manage your tension over time through exercise, dietary changes, and meditation. This reduction in stress helps not only brain fog, but overall mental and physical health.

Medication

Many medications, both over-the-counter and prescription, have brain fog as a side effect. If these medications are taken infrequently, the brain fog may only be a temporary issue to be worked through. However, with long-term medications it's advisable to have a discussion with your doctor regarding the effect on your brain. Sometimes there are alternative medications or other changes that will alleviate this side effect.

Depression and Anxiety

Both depression and anxiety are associated with impaired cognitive function, memory, attention, and executive function (how your brain and body prioritize their functions). This impairment is linked to low energy and loss of motivation. This is the kind of brain fog where there may just be too much to think about and your mind shuts down under the pressure. Talk to your healthcare provider about treatment options if you're struggling with anxiety or depression.

Thyroid Disorders

If you feel you're tired all the time, that you lack mental clarity and focus, or have frequent mood swings, the root of these symptoms can be a thyroid disorder. The thyroid is a butterfly-shaped gland located in the front of your neck that is responsible for producing hormones that control bodily functions from breathing to heart rate, and metabolism to menstrual cycles. When the thyroid doesn't work correctly by producing too much hormone (hyperthyroidism) or too little (hypothyroidism), it can cripple both the body and the brain. This particularly true when it comes to Hashimoto's thyroiditis, an autoimmune disorder in which your immune system attacks your thyroid gland and prevents it from producing the necessary hormones, creating inflammation and increased stress throughout the body. A blood test can be performed to test the function of the thyroid so proper treatment can be determined.

Heavy Metal Exposure

We are exposed to metals every day in our lives, in sources like food, beauty products, and even the fillings in our teeth. Much of this exposure is harmless or even helpful to the function of the body and the brain. We need trace elements and metals to create energy and strengthen our bones and muscles. However, some metals are a problem, especially when they build up in our systems. The most common problematic metals are those classed as heavy metals, including mercury, lead, aluminum, arsenic, cesium, and thallium. Limited exposure or consumption of these metals don't lead to toxicity, but the accumulation from chronic exposure can lead to hormonal imbalance, immune dysfunction, brain fog, fatigue, and high blood pressure. High levels of heavy metals in water supplies have also been linked to learning disabilities and dysfunction in children. This exposure can be lessened by being aware of the mineral content of your water and choosing foods in their natural forms, free from processing.

What is a Brain Detox?

A brain cleanse or detox is a process to help in protecting you against neurodegenerative diseases and decreasing the symptoms related to poor functioning of the brain.

Typically, people go through a brain detox in order to manage symptoms such as:

- Brain fog
- Anxiety
- Depression
- Fatigue
- Memory loss
- Addictions
- Brain stroke and injury

The key to a brain detox is to focus on targeting and treating the root cause of these chronic illnesses and restore your wellness. When you start a brain detox, it's recommended that you prioritize sleep, consume an anti-inflammatory diet, exercise, and take specific supplements that support the functioning of your brain.

When you try a new detox, it's always a good idea to take it one step at a time. You didn't get where you are overnight, and detoxing and removing stress from body and mind won't happen overnight either. Choose to add one or two good changes at a time and set realistic, measurable goals so you can see your success.

If you're interested in delving further into the benefits brain detox, you might be interested in my other book in the Things We Need To Do series, Detox Our Brain.

What Does a Mental Detox Look Like?

A mental detox is created by making changes in your life-style that relieve stress and balance both your body and your brain. You can start by consuming proper nutrient-rich foods, getting plenty of sleep, exercising, and resetting your body overall. Let's take a look at each of these changes to understand how to detox our brains better.

Anti-Inflammatory Diet

Diet plays a crucial role when it comes to managing your gut-brain connection and cognitive health. Your brain requires a constant supply of nutrients to be at its best. These nutrients include antioxidants, proteins, omega-3 fatty acids, healthy fats, and the all-important vitamins and minerals. Healthy brain foods fight against free radical damage and boost your intake of nutrients.

Types of foods you may want to include in your mental detox diet include those rich in antioxidants which have anti-carcinogenic and anti-inflammatory effects, such as:

- Seeds and nuts
- Vegetables and fruits that are rich in bioflavonoids, like beets, leafy vegetables, bell peppers, broccoli, oranges, and berries
- Beans and legumes which are high in fiber and iron
- Spices and herbs like turmeric, rosemary, garlic, and ginger
- Probiotic, fermented foods such as yogurt, kimchi, kefir, and sauerkraut
- Pastured poultry and free-range eggs
- Wild-caught fish
- Healthy fats like olive oil, avocados, grass-fed butter, and coconut oil
- Grass-fed meats
- Complex carbohydrates such as sweet potatoes and whole grains with minimal processing
- Foods rich in vitamin C, copper, and manganese, like berries, mushrooms, citrus fruits, leafy greens, algae, spirulina, and organ meats

Apart from consuming a healthy diet, you will want to avoid foods that increase inflammation, oxidative stress, and autoimmune reactions. Included in this list are processed meats, added sugars, trans fats and vegetable oils, and highly processed foods, generally. Proper hydration is also critical to support these healthy changes. Don't forget to drink plenty of water!

Exercise

Exercise is a great way to enhance lymphatic activity and stimulate your digestive system as well as encouraging natural detoxification. It also plays a role in increasing your brain's plasticity, a critical part of memory and learning. Exercise also helps you cope with stress, have more energy, and sleep deeply.

Most adults should aim for a minimum of 30 minutes of moderate exercise every day, which can also be separated into shorter sessions. These workouts increase the flow of highly oxygenated blood to your brain which supports mitochondrial function and helps to prevent dementia.

You can make things challenging and interesting for you and your body by trying out different workouts like walking, running, cycling, weightlifting, Pilates, yoga, swimming, etc. Always consult with a doctor before starting a new exercise regime and work within your physical limitations.

Reduce Toxin Exposure

While it might not sound realistic, or even possible, to avoid the toxins and chemicals found in nearly every aspect of our lives, it's a good idea to try to reduce your exposure to these contaminants as much as you can. Opt for buying organic, minimally processed foods and use organic products such as deodorants and shampoos when possible. Toxins are found everywhere and in most of the products we use in our daily lives. It's important to acknowledge this and make good choices where you can.

Feed Your Brain

Your brain, like many of your other internal organs, is made up of a lot of protein and fat. So, does it make sense that most modern diets are low in both protein and good fat? Not really. Your brain does not benefit from sugary, processed foods. Stick to fruits, vegetables, plenty of protein, and good fats. You can also include omega-3 fatty acids, antioxidants, and coenzyme Q10 to boost your mental health and feed your brain.

Consider Taking Supplements

You may consider supporting your body's natural detoxing ability by consuming supplements, nootropics (cognition enhancers), and adaptogenic herbs that assist with nourishing your kidneys, liver, gut, and brain. These include:

- L-glutamine to support the gastrointestinal tract
- Green tea extracts for a boost of energy and antioxidants
- Milk thistle to support the liver
- Vitamin C to support the immune system
- NAD+ to support mitochondria
- Probiotics to maintain healthy gut flora and support the gut in general
- Medicinal mushrooms to support the immune system

Rest Your Digestive System

In the dieting world intermittent fasting has become all the rage. This type of diet restricts calories and builds a schedule around your eating that can lead to weight loss. However, this isn't the only benefit of cutting back on the calories and spacing your meals out. Fasting promotes neurological health and decreases the likelihood of developing neurodegenerative diseases.

You don't need to jump into intermittent fasting all at once. Start by extending the time between your dinner and your breakfast the next day. Aim for a minimum of 12 hours between these two meals and let your gut rest. This promotes ketogenesis — the body burning fat instead of fast carbs — which also stimulates brain regeneration.

Prioritize Sleep

Sleep plays an important role when it comes to making healthy decisions. When you don't get enough sleep, you're likely to have increased cravings for junk food and other stimulants. Getting enough sleep every night is one of the best ways to support your brain's natural process of detoxification.

Most adults require around seven to nine hours of sleep every night to operate at their best.

Key Takeaways

When your gut health is poor, it compromises your brain health. A good brain and body detox helps reduce brain fog so you can concentrate and be your best you.

6

Drink More of This

Detox drinks have gained popularity over the past few years for to preventing toxic overload and related health problems.

When you consume detox drinks regularly, it helps with weight loss, eases digestion, moves material through the intestines, and boosts your metabolism. These detox drinks also enhance the functioning of the liver, improve the condition of your skin and hair, and support better sleep.

One potential drawback with detoxing, especially when it comes to what you drink, is the need to give up alcohol and coffee, which can, of course, be a difficult process. But for the best results, it's important that you give them both up while you are on your detox diet, and very possibly beyond. This is easier if it's a gradual process. Removing caffeine and alcohol from your diet may well cause headaches and discomfort at first, but this will pass as you replace these drinks with more water and detox drinks.

Water is an essential component to healthy living and a natural detox drink. Most Americans don't drink nearly enough water on a daily basis. It's recommended that you consume a minimum of two to four cups of water per day, although six to eight is usually better, depending on your personal health. Normally, the color of your urine will give you a good indication of how hydrated you are. The darker it is, the more water you need to drink, so you should be aiming for a very pale yellow. Consuming water helps:

- Prevent constipation
- Carry oxygen and nutrients to your cells
- Improve digestion
- Flush bacteria out from your bladder

Water to Prevent Dehydration

Not only is water our primary detox drink, but it's also essential for our very survival. So, let's look at the benefits of H2O in a little more depth.

Benefits of Drinking Water

Water helps to keep all the systems in your body functioning at their best. The water you drink performs several important tasks, including:

- Prevent constipation in your body
- Aid digestion
- Carry oxygen and nutrients to your cells
- Stabilize your heartbeats
- Flush bacteria out of your bladder
- Protect your tissues and organs

- Cushion your joints
- Normalize blood pressure
- Maintain electrolyte balance
- Regulate your body temperature

You need to feed your body enough water and other fluids to carry out these tasks. If you don't drink enough water, you will become dehydrated, which — in extreme cases — will eventually lead to death. Some warning signs of dehydration include low blood pressure, confusion, weakness, dizziness, and dark-colored urine.

How Much Water Should You Drink Each Day?

There is no one-size-fits-all rule when it comes to how much water you should drink in a day. We've talked about the general rule of dividing your weight in pounds by two and drinking that many ounces of water, but water needs do vary from one person to the other. For example, if you're sweating because of exercise or a hot environment, or if you have a health condition like liver, heart, or kidney problems, you will need to drink more water. Some medications, like antidepressants, opiate medications, and non-steroidal anti-inflammatory drugs (NSAIDs) can cause water retention which can only be eased by drinking more water. Learn to listen to your body and keep that water bottle handy.

Tips to Avoid Dehydration

Of course, it's not just plain water that helps you stay hydrated. All beverages that contain water add to your daily water needs.

However, it's usually best to choose water over any other drink, particularly for detox purposes. Sugary drinks lead to inflammation and weight gain, increasing your risk of developing diseases like diabetes. Too much caffeine can keep you from getting enough sleep and make you anxious, and your alcohol intake should be no more than one or two drinks per day.

To prevent dehydration, be sure to drink fluids gradually throughout the day. You can do this easily by having water with every meal, with your medicines, and by keeping it on hand at all times in a reusable water bottle so that you can keep sipping all day.

If you'd like to make your water intake a little more interesting and appetizing, consider adding cucumber or lemon, which is an excellent detoxifier.

Benefits of Lemon Detox Water

Adding lemon to water increases the flavor, but it also has additional detoxification properties. Let's take a look at how lemon water can be a beneficial part of your detox diet.

Promotes Hydration

We've already touched on all the reasons to stay properly hydrated, but many people complain that water, which tastes of nothing, is boring. Lemon water has more flavor, which can make it more palatable and encourage you to reach your daily drinking goals.

Supports Weight Loss

Drinking water also helps to support healthy weight loss because it starts the process of breaking down body fat. It's common when you think you're hungry that you're actually dehydrated and misinterpreting the hunger signal from your body. Also, drinking more water is associated with eating less food. Lemon water contains antioxidants that improve your insulin response so that less food is stored as fat and sugar spikes aren't as significant — all good things when it comes to weight loss and maintenance.

Great Source of Vitamin C

Citrus fruits are some of the best sources of vitamin C. Adding lemon to your water is an easy way to increase your vitamin C intake and support your immune system.

Aids Digestion

Many people find consuming lemon water helps to treat or prevent constipation. When you drink warm lemon water just after waking up in the morning, it hydrates your stomach and gut and gets your digestive system going.

How Lemon Water Helps Detox

Lemon water does not detox the body entirely. If you want to accomplish a full detox, you need to get rid of the toxins from your gastrointestinal tract, and to carry out this process, your body needs fiber. Lemons are not rich in fiber, but they are high in the vitamin C that boosts your immune system. Lemon water helps flush out toxins from your body and cleanse the liver, but this process is made even more effective when you also consume high-fiber fruits and vegetables.

Detox Water Recipes for De-Bloating and Boosting Your Metabolism

Water infused with fruits, vegetables, or herbs might not get rid of all the evils in your system, but they certainly help to kick-start your metabolism, deliver nutrients to your body in the most natural possible way, and support your liver. Several detox waters are also high in natural antioxidants that can reverse cell damage. The increased consumption of water along with anti-inflammatory ingredients helps you become de-bloated naturally.

Let's look at some detox water recipes and how they help your body. Keep in mind you should always use natural, organic ingredients when you can. Fresh herbs, fruits, and vegetables are much better than those that have been processed for long storage.

Plain Water

Ingredients:

- Water (preferably filtered)

Benefits to your body

Promotes the detoxification process, improves blood circulation, reduces inflammation, facilitates digestion, relieves constipation, boosts energy, curbs your hunger between meals, decreases sugar cravings, and makes your skin glow.

Liver-Loving Water

Ingredients:

- 1 liter water (about 33.8 oz)
- 2 tablespoons fresh turmeric juice
- 2 dropperfuls burdock tincture
- 3–4 slices of lemon

Benefits to your body

The human liver is known to be a powerhouse detox factory since it detoxifies hormones and toxins and facilitates important metabolic processes. Burdock in this water improves the elimination process and liver function, while turmeric has strong anti-inflammatory properties. Lemon improves the natural detoxification process. This detox water is a great choice to support a healthy liver.

Body-Cooling Cucumber Water

Ingredients:

- 1 sliced cucumber
- 1 sliced lime
- Pinch of Himalayan salt
- 4 cups alkaline water

Directions:

If you have limited time, an infused detox water such as this can be thrown together in a minute. You just need to add all the ingredients to a large pitcher and keep it in your refrigerator so it's always on hand.

Benefits to your body

The ingredients in this water contain large amounts of vitamin A and vitamin C. This drink also contains potassium and silica, both vital minerals for the body which help prevent muscle spasms and pain.

Cucumber, Mint, and Lemon Water

Ingredients:

- 1 lemon
- ½ cucumber
- A few mint leaves
- 2 liters water

Directions:

Wash and slice the lemon and cucumber and rinse the mint leaves. Place both lemon and cucumber into a water jug. Fill the jug with water, mix the ingredients together, and leave it overnight in the fridge to steep. You can top off the jug with water for a couple of days until the flavor dissipates, then you need to begin again.

Benefits to your body

This energizing and refreshing detox water is rich in antioxidants thanks to vitamin A from the mint and vitamin C from the lemon. Lemon interacts positively with the enzymes in your body and stimulates gastric juices, assists the liver to produce enzymes, cleanses the blood and arteries, and releases toxins. Lemon also increases the body's ability to absorb minerals, improve digestion, and reduce inflammation. The mint in the water provides anti-inflammatory properties and aids in digestion. Additionally, the aroma of the lemon awakens your senses and makes you feel more energized.

Watermelon and Mint Refresher

Ingredients:

- 1 cup cubed watermelon
- 1 handful of fresh mint leaves
- 4 cups alkaline water

Directions:

Lightly crush watermelon cubes and add to a jug with mint leaves. Cover with water and allow to steep.

Benefits to your body

Watermelon is rich in potassium, a mineral that supports several organs. This includes the kidneys, which are responsible for flushing out toxins from your system.

Ginger Mint Water

Ingredients:

- 1 thinly sliced cucumber
- 2 lemon or lime wedges
- 10–12 fresh mint leaves
- 2 inches freshly peeled ginger root
- Pinch of Himalayan salt
- Water

Directions:

Combine cucumber and citrus in a jug. Gently bruise mint leaves and lightly crush ginger root, then add to the cucumber and citrus mixture. Add salt and water. Allow to steep and keep in the refrigerator.

Benefits to your body

Ginger is a proven digestive aid that reduces intestinal discomfort and gas, helps prevent bad bacteria from entering the gut, and eases stomach ulcers. Ginger also has potent anti-inflammatory components that reduce inflammation wherever it is found.

Ginger can relieve nausea and reduces blood insulin levels that aid in weight management. Fresh ginger soothes a sore throat and may help prevent the common cold. The anti-inflammatory properties of ginger reduce pain and soothes inflammation in your throat that occurs due to any kind of infection.

Classic Berry-Infused Water

Ingredients:

- 2 cleaned and sliced strawberries
- 4 cleaned and halved red raspberries
- 6 cleaned and halved blueberries
- 4 cleaned and halved black raspberries

Directions:

Fill a 24-ounce (about 700 ml) jug with ice cubes and add all ingredients. Fill the jug with water. Soak for a minimum of four hours before you drink it.

Benefits to your body

This berry-infused drink is a great way to get your water in while enjoying a refreshing and flavorful drink. Berries are packed with antioxidants, vitamins, and minerals, plus they are low on the glycemic index, meaning they won't cause a spike in your blood sugar. Blueberries and black raspberries, in particular, consist of a flavonoid known as anthocyanin, a plant compound that contains powerful antioxidants.

Teas for Detox

If you love tea, there are some great herbal teas for detox and battling bloat. Low-caffeine or entirely caffeine-free teas like parsley, ginger, or dandelion root are great options when you want to have a light and healthy detox. It's advised that you drink these teas at least twice a day, once before breakfast and once before dinner, so they can assist your digestive system. Make sure that you drink them along with your meals and not as a meal replacement.

Dandelion Tea

One of the natural ways you eliminate toxins from your body is by urinating, and the dandelion root in this tea promotes urination. It is a great digestive aid that cleans your kidneys and liver.

Milk Thistle

Milk thistle might seem a strange brew since it is called milk, but it doesn't contain any dairy components. The milk in the tea is sourced by crushing cuttings from the milk thistle plant. This milk from the plant reduces inflammation and liver damage and facilitates cell repair.

Fennel Tea

When we talk about Ayurvedic medicine, fennel is a go-to since it impacts the digestive system, which is the foundation of health in Ayurveda. Fennel tea is used therapeutically for stimulating digestive functions and appetite. It helps to relieve constipation and relaxes your digestive muscles, allowing your body to get rid of the toxins in your body more easily.

Lemongrass Rooibos Tea

The reddish-brown rooibos tea is derived from the South African red bush's fermented leaves. These leaves are known for their strong antioxidant properties that make them ideal for detoxifying your body. This tea is delicious, and the addition of lemongrass brings a bright flavor and powerful anti-inflammatory properties.

Turmeric Ginger Tea

The active ingredient in turmeric, curcumin, helps the enzymes in your body to eliminate toxins while the abundance of antioxidants aid in repairing liver cells. Turmeric also supports your liver in disposing of metals and boosts the production of bile.

Cilantro or Parsley Tea

Of course, all teas that you make will contain water, which is, in itself, a powerful detoxing agent. But when you make teas with herbs that are natural diuretics, it doubles the benefits.

Cilantro and parsley facilitate water elimination and nourishing your kidneys and other detox organs.

Green Tea

For several years, green tea has been considered a powerful health elixir, and with good reason. Green tea is derived from young tea leaves and contain a potent and powerful antioxidant known as epigallocatechin-3-gallate (EGCG), which protects your liver against diseases and cancerous growths. Green tea also contains L-theanine, an amino acid used to produce the vital antioxidant, glutathione.

Smoothies for Detox

While water and other light detox drinks are a great go-to for hydration and taking care of your body, you might also want to consider drinking smoothies as part of your detox. Smoothies allow you to add calories, fiber, and other vitamins and nutrients to your diet, however, how healthy your smoothie depends on the kind of ingredients you blend. When considering a smoothie, avoid added sugars and sodium, or processed ingredients with artificial sugars or preservatives.

Green Smoothies

A green smoothie made from beets, carrots, spinach, kale, parsley, celery, turnip, and cloves contains amazing nutrients for your body and no salt, fat, or processed sugar.

You might find a few of these ingredients in the smoothie overpowering. But you can replace them with ingredients that have similar nutrient contents and work your way up to a smoothie with all the ingredients.

Fruit Smoothies

Fruits are a delicious, sweet base for a smoothie, but should be used in moderation as fruit sugars can increase calorie counts and trigger blood sugar spikes — although they are generally milder than spikes caused by processed sugars and simple carbohydrates. Using the whole fruit increases the fiber in your smoothie, making a drink that is healthier than the juice alone.

You can also add protein to your fruit smoothie by adding yogurt. Unflavored Greek yogurt contains about 9 grams of protein per 100 grams and gives a smoothie a rich creaminess.

Combinations

Many people enjoy combining both vegetables and fruits in their smoothies. This is the best way to make veggie smoothies taste amazing or not overload your fruit smoothie with too much sugar.

If you're feeling adventurous, you can consider adding nuts and seeds, which make for great sources of fiber, protein, and fatty acids. Try adding chia or flax seeds to give a boost to the omega-3 content in your smoothie.

You can also add oats or bran fiber to thicken your smoothie. When you like the taste and texture of a smoothie you will be encouraged to drink it more often. Experiment with fresh, organic ingredients to figure out what suits you and your body the best.

Key Takeaways

Daily hydration is necessary for the best function of your brain and body. There are lots of great ways to fill your hydration needs with water infusions, teas, and smoothies. These drinks are not only tasty but a necessary aspect of detox and part of a healthy diet. Adding whole fruits, vegetables, and whole grains to your drinks is an easy way to increase your consumption of these health-friendly foods.

These hydrating drinks are best when included in a diet full of fresh fruits and vegetables, fiber-rich foods, and healthy proteins. Eating these things in combination and moderation will support and promote your body's natural detoxification process.

Substance Abuse, Recovery and Detox

A busing substances like drugs and alcohol often result in your making poor diet choices, such as skipping meals, late-night snacking, and choosing junk food. When you abuse drugs, it can keep your body from receiving the nutrients it requires from the food you eat. Abusing drugs also reduces your daily nutrition intake and makes a proper diet and detox even more important for your full recovery.

Although detox withdrawal symptoms differ from one substance to another, one of the most common symptoms is lack of appetite, which is generally accompanied by vomiting and nausea. When you are strong enough to keep liquids and food down again, it's important that you feed your body with proper nutrients.

Nutritional Impact of Alcohol and Drugs

Both alcohol and drugs impact how your body's basic functions work. Alcohol impairs your body's digestive enzymes and how it controls glucose levels. Abusing opioids results in slower digestion and, in turn, constipation. Several stimulants result in eating disorders and have a multitude of negative side effects, such as anxiety, insomnia, and malnutrition.

What Your Body Actually Needs

When you're partaking of drugs or alcohol, it creates nutritional deficiencies. Your body's increased nutritional needs depend on the kind of substance you use. Let's discuss some common substances and what you can eat for each.

Alcohol Recovery Foods

Alcohol is a substance that is easily accessed but is very damaging to the body. It contains a lot of empty calories — even more so when it's served in cocktails or other heavy drinks.

Regular alcohol consumption leads to deficiencies in vitamin B6, folic acid, and thiamine. Individuals who drink alcohol frequently also have an imbalance of electrolytes, protein, and fluids. All this results in the liver and pancreas having to work harder, causing organ damage, high blood pressure, and — in extreme cases — seizures. When you take good multivitamins, you can combat some of the deficiencies that occur with alcoholism.

Women who have been hard drinkers for some time can benefit from calcium supplements, since they can be at a higher risk of developing osteoporosis. If you're recovering from alcoholism, you will need to consume a healthy diet that would help you recover from malnutrition. Therefore, it's important to drink plenty of water and to eat a diet that has a good general balance of grains, vegetables, fruit and lean protein. Good choices for addressing vitamin and mineral deficiencies are:

- White rice and egg noodles, which are rich in thiamine
- Lean meat and fish, especially tuna and salmon
- Kale, cabbage, brussels sprouts and broccoli
- Legumes like kidney beans and chickpeas
- Bananas, oranges, papaya and cantaloupe

Opioid Addiction Foods

Opioids, such as heroin and Oxycontin, are very hard on the digestive system. If you're addicted to these substances, you will likely deal with diarrhea, nausea, constipation, and vomiting. This situation leads to electrolyte imbalances in your body, so you should focus on a diet that is rich in fiber to decrease gastrointestinal trouble and regulate the electrolyte imbalance. Some foods that you can eat that are high in fiber are:

- Whole grains such as bulgur wheat, barley, and rye
- Vegetables such as spinach, broccoli, and lima beans
- Beans such as lentils, black beans, and navy beans

Marijuana Use Foods

Unlike other drugs, marijuana tends to increase your appetite, generating the many jokes about someone having the munchies after using marijuana. However, this appetite increase is usually in the form of cravings that mean you end up eating foods that are high in sugar, sodium, and fat. When you are on your detox, your focus must be on the reduced calorie intake and determining that perfect balance with foods that will help nourish your body. Remember to drink plenty of water and keep snacks of fruits and vegetables on hand. In particular, nuts can be a good snack to satisfy these cravings, such as almonds, cashews and macadamias.

Stimulant Addiction Foods

Stimulants like methamphetamine and cocaine provide you with a high feeling that reduces your appetite and the need for sleep. Due to this, your body will require fluids to fight dehydration. You might need to increase your healthy caloric intake to replace the energy that you lose. Staying awake for a prolonged period is extremely bad for your health and causes a number of physical and mental problems. Heavy stimulant abuse can even lead to permanent damage to your memory.

Why Junk Food Doesn't Work Against Addiction

Whether you are a habitual drug user or more a social dabbler, there are many reasons why you should opt for foods that are rich in nutrients in order to support your health in general. This is especially true when you are recovering from an addiction or are on long-term prescription medication, such as in the case of chronic disease patients. Take a look at these reasons below.

Your Body Requires Nutrients for Healing

When you are, or have been, relying on alcohol or drugs, it can be difficult for you to recognize when you have nutrition deficiencies. When you provide your body with appropriate nutrients, such as B-vitamins and Omega-3 fatty acids, it gives you fuel to deal with withdrawal symptoms and overall improved energy. As you bring your body into a better state of health, it will be much easier for you to ignore your cravings and make better dietary choices.

Your Body Requires Fiber to Function Well

Taking multivitamins will replace some of the nutrients that you need in when you're eating poorly, but they will not sustain you over the long term. For that reason, it's important to consume a lot of fruits, vegetables, and whole grains. Not only will the fiber content in them keep your digestive system functioning properly, but it will also help in regulating your blood sugar levels. This means that you will experience less irritability and fewer mood swings. This too will help with cravings for the substances you are trying to avoid as well as the sugars and heavy fats that slow you down.

You Don't Want to Replace Your Addiction

While recovering, many people use caffeine and sugar to keep themselves alert and awake. However, over a period, your brain will start expecting all food to taste sweet, so the healthier foods will not taste as good as the sweet ones. Consuming high-sugar foods will become another problem for you if you use sugar to substitute your addiction.

Detox Food and Dieting Practices

So, what should you be eating as part your addiction recovery? Most of the detox foods we have talked about fit the bill perfectly to assist in your recovery and make you healthier in your body and your mind.

Fruits

Fruits, just like vegetables, consist of phytonutrients that provide you with immense health benefits. According to USDA dietary guidelines, if you are a healthy adult, you should consume about 1.5 to 2 cups of fruit every day. And that's whole fruits, not fruit juices.

You can select from whole fruits, either fresh or frozen, which can include:

- Apples
- Grapes
- Cherries
- Apricots
- Cantaloupe
- Blueberries
- Blackberries
- Cranberries
- Figs
- Oranges
- Grapefruit
- Mango
- Melon
- Limes
- Guava

- Watermelon
- Strawberries
- Tangerines
- Plums
- Peaches
- Papayas
- Pears
- Pomegranates
- Prunes
- Kiwis
- Loganberries

Whole Grains and Complex Carbs

Every person has their own group of go-to carbs, which is often bread, potatoes, and pasta. While these can be healthy choices, especially when they are made from whole grains and the crust and/or skins are also consumed, why not experimenting with other healthy sources of complex carbs and whole grains as well? Some of these options may be familiar to you, while others could be a new food experience.

- Oats
- Quinoa
- Tapioca
- Arrowroot
- Buckwheat
- Amaranth
- Brown rice
- Wild rice
- Barley
- Millet

- Freekeh
- Farro
- Sweet potato or yams
- Teff
- Winter squash – spaghetti squash, acorn squash and butternut squash among others

It's best to eat unrefined whole grains, but you can also find benefits in consuming products that have them as an ingredient. These can include glass noodles, buckwheat soba noodles, brown rice pasta, mung bean noodles, rice crackers, kelp noodles, rice bran, quinoa flakes, shirataki noodles, and gluten-free bread. Not only are these whole grains great sources of fiber and energy, but experimenting with different types keeps your diet interesting and therefore easier to stick with.

Beans and Legumes

Beans and legumes are rich in iron, protein, and fiber to make you feel full and satisfied. They are great in dishes or as a side and are complimented by herbs and spices. They are also very varied, with plenty of choice. You can try:

- Lentils - green, yellow, brown, red, du Puy, or French
- Green peas and split yellow peas
- Other beans and legumes like chickpeas, black-eyed peas, lima beans, kidney beans, pinto beans, red beans, white beans, cannellini, and adzuki

Fats

During your detox, make sure that you avoid trans fats and consume only healthy fats that are sourced from raw nuts, seeds, avocado, and seed and nut butters. Try some of the following to add crunch to a dish along with fats that are good for your internal organs.

- Cashews
- Almonds
- Pistachios
- Hazelnuts
- Walnuts
- Chia seeds
- Brazil nuts
- Coconut
- Flax seeds
- Macadamia nuts
- Help nuts, hemp seeds, hemp hearts
- Pine nuts
- Sesame seeds
- Sunflower seeds
- Pumpkin seeds
- Poppy seeds
- Pecans
- Seed and nut butter, like almond butter, cashew nut butter, and tahini
- Pine nuts

Also, when you're cooking with oil, make sure that you use high-quality, unrefined, and cold-pressed oils such as:

- Almond oil
- Coconut oil
- Olive oil
- Sunflower oil
- Hazelnut oil
- Flax oil
- Avocado oil
- Hemp oil
- Safflower oil
- Walnut oil
- Pumpkin oil

Some of these oils have low smoking points so be sure to heat them gently. Any of these oils work well in vinaigrettes or other dressings to go with dark leafy greens or other vegetables.

Staying Hydrated to Fend off Withdrawal and Cravings

You can limit your caffeine and alcohol intake by swapping them for herbal, white, or green tea and unsweetened, flavored waters. Here are some beverage options that you can choose from.

- Lemon water
- Coconut water
- Seltzer or mineral water
- Infused water or detox water
- Unsweetened kombucha
- True teas, like white tea and green tea
- Herbal teas like ginger tea, rooibos tea, and cinnamon tea

- Plant-based milk like almond milk, rice milk, oat milk, and hemp milk
- Unsweetened juice that is made from vegetables and fruits

If you're not able to give up on your morning coffee, try to limit it to just one 8-ounce cup. Also, make sure that you avoid any added sweeteners.

Condiments

Spices, fresh herbs, and dried herbs make any meal even more flavorful without the addition of salt or sugar. Many herbs and spices also have anti-inflammatory properties and support body health. Try topping your meals with chopped fresh herbs like cilantro, basil, mint, oregano, parsley, thyme, rosemary, chives, dill, sage, or tarragon.

Examples of spices that you can add while cooking include cardamom, cinnamon, coriander, cloves, nutmeg, tamarind, cumin, turmeric, allspice, caraway seeds, or anise. These are even tastier if you purchase the spice whole and grind it yourself.

Raw or fresh ginger and garlic make your meals instantly more interesting and flavorful. You can also consider the following ingredients and condiments as being good options when you are detoxing:

- Baking powder or baking soda
- Coconut amino acids
- Sea salt
- Olives
- Mustard

- Limes and lemons
- Cacao nibs and cacao powder
- Carob powder
- Fish sauce
- Nama shoyu
- Nutritional yeast
- Wheat-free tamari
- Miso
- Vinegar such as apple cider vinegar, coconut, balsamic, white or red wine

Sugars and Other Sweeteners

It's very positive for your body when you limit your overall intake of sugar and sweets from all possible sources. However, if you are going to use a sweetener, make sure that you choose a natural source like:

- Honey
- Stevia
- Maple syrup
- Coconut nectar
- Brown rice syrup
- Fruit jam – low or no sugar
- Monk fruit
- Dried fruit
- Blackstrap molasses

For your desserts, you can choose fresh, whole fruits, or try out frozen puddings and desserts that are made from nuts, yogurt, milk, and fruits.

Animal Protein

There is a lot of debate when it comes to the inclusion of animal protein in detox diets. In general, lean proteins are good building blocks for the body and the Omega-3 fatty acids from fish are heart healthy. If you wish to consume animal protein, you can consider the following options:

- Lamb
- Organic turkey
- Organic chicken
- Sardines and anchovies
- Wild game like buffalo, ostrich, bison, quail, pheasant, and venison
- Wild, cold-water fishes like Alaskan salmon

You're Not Craving Drugs, You're Just Hungry

Most of the people who have used drugs or alcohol for a long time can forget how it feels to be hungry. Once their bodies start to recover, these feelings can come back all at once. It's recommended that you stay on a regular meal schedule when you are detoxing, and even after you are done detoxing. This will teach your body when it can expect food and help you in keeping the hunger cravings under check so that you don't overeat or be tempted by cravings.

Learn to Cook a Few Meals

You don't need to master the art of cooking to cook healthy foods. However, learning to cook even just a few basic, healthy meals can be very satisfying and a good way to raise your nutrition levels. You can find a multitude of recipes and tutorials online. You can also consider investing in a good slow cooker or counter-top pressure cooker. This equipment can make cooking easy because you simply toss in all the ingredients, switch the machine on, and let it cook. After a few hours – sometimes minutes, in the case of the pressure cooker! — you will have your hot meal ready. It's easier to eat well when you have healthy, satisfying options on hand.

Healthy Habits to Include with Your Detox Diet

Using detox and a healthy diet is a huge step forward in your recovery or maintenance process, but it's only the first step. There are other good habits you can cultivate that will support you in becoming a healthier version of yourself.

Say No to Cigarettes

Not only do cigarettes contain harmful tars and carcino-gens, but they also play a crucial role as an addiction trigger for harder drugs. Smoking can also prompt cravings for sugars and fatty foods, so it's easy to see how removing this habit will quickly improve your overall health.

Stay Positive

Not every situation can be fixed with a positive attitude, but there is some truth to the idea of "mind over matter". Facing stressful situations and challenges with a positive atti-tude helps mitigate the stress responses in the mind and the body.

Exercise

Exercising, even light exercise like walking, is beneficial for you both physically and mentally. When you exercise you support your natural detoxification, your body burns fat, strengthens your muscles and heart, and your brain produces endorphins. Endorphins are chemicals in the body that bring you feelings of contentment, help balance your mood, and strengthen your response to stress.

Get Proper Sleep

Sleeping enough is one of the most important elements to your health and mental well-being. When you sleep you're giving your body time to recharge and recover and your mind time to process information and rest. When you don't get enough sleep, it's difficult for your systems to perform their day-to-day functions.

Key Takeaways

Participating in a detox diet as part of rehabilitation from drug and alcohol use can be very positive. It's important that you understand the substances you have been taking and the effects they have on the body and what foods and drinks will help to undo the damage that has been done to your body.

8

Fasting as Part of Detox

W e've mentioned intermittent fasting as part of a
detox diet earlier in this volume, but in this chapter, we'll go into more details as to why fasting works and
what you can expect.

People have participated in fasting over centuries, whether
for religious purposes or out of necessity.

Fasting refers to the willing reduction or absence from all or
some foods, liquids, or even both, over a specific period of
time. Though sometimes it's referred to as depriving,
unhealthy, or simply reserved for religious reasons, fasting
for a short time can offer you significant health benefits. As
a part of a healthy diet, fasting gives your body the opportunity to rest and recover. It's similar to having a good
night's sleep and letting yourself start fresh the next
morning.

Fasting is now widely accepted as a beneficial way to prevent disease and manage weight. At the same time, it's essential that you fast in healthy ways.

Typically, most fasts are conducted over a period of 24 to 72 hours.

On the other hand, the eating pattern known as intermittent fasting consists of shifts between periods of fasting and eating that range from a few hours to even a few days.

While fasting is generally a healthy addition to a detox diet, there are situations where you wouldn't want to follow this type of eating regime, including when you're pregnant, if you have suffered from an eating disorder in the past or if you're doing any extreme exercise. The point of fasting as part of your diet is to work with your body's natural rhythms for better health, not to stop eating altogether.

The Science of Fasting

Fasting helps your body detox by forcing cells into bodily processes that don't get stimulated when you continually fuel your body with food. When you fast, your body doesn't have access to glucose, so that forces the cells to resort to other materials and sources for producing energy. The end result is that your body starts the process of gluconeogenesis, which enables your body to produce its own sugar. Your liver converts non-carbohydrate materials, such as amino acids, fats, and lactate into glucose. Since your body conserves energy when you're fasting, your basal metabolic rate, which refers to the amount of energy your body burns at rest, becomes more efficient. This lowers your blood pressure and heart rate.

Ketosis is another process that occurs in the latter part of your fasting cycle. It refers to the point when your body burns stored fat and uses it as its primary source of energy. This is an ideal way to lose weight and balance your blood sugar levels. Ketosis fasting should be carefully monitored, though. Staying in this state for short periods of time burns stored fat, but if it goes on too long there can be loss of lean muscle mass instead.

Fasting puts your body under some stress, making your cells adapt, thereby enhancing their coping abilities. In simpler words, your cells become stronger, making your body stronger. This process is very similar to what happens when you stress your cardiovascular system and muscles while exercising. However, it's important to remember that as with exercise, periods of stressing and strengthening your cells should be followed by rest and recovery. For this reason, it's recommended that your fasting be taken in cycles to give your body everything that it needs to maintain your health.

Benefits of Fasting

If you're thinking that giving your body regular breaks from food will aid in weight loss, research suggests that you're right! However, fasting comes with other health benefits as well. This is what science has to say about it.

Fasting Helps You Lose Weight

Fasting on alternate days has been proven to be as efficient for weight loss as a traditional low-calorie diet. You consume fewer calories between your periods of fasting, which also has a positive effect on your blood sugar levels and fat burning.

A review written in 2015 concluded that when you fast for an entire day each week, it helps in shedding up to 6 percent of your total body fat in just about 12 weeks (Tinsley & La Bounty, 2015).

However, how you break the fast matters as well. If you break your fast with a diet of junk food, fried food, and processed carbs you won't be able to maintain any of the healthy benefits of fasting. Fasting needs to be part of a healthy lifestyle, not just a quick weight loss scheme to drop a few pounds for a holiday party.

Helps Keep Blood Sugar Levels Steady

When you fast, your body starts to depend more on burning fats rather than carbohydrates to produce power. When your body isn't burning carbohydrates your blood sugar levels remain lower. This leads to a decrease in the production of insulin and stabilizes blood sugar spikes.

Intermittent fasting can also reduce insulin resistance. Because your body isn't taking in as many simple sugars and doesn't overproduce insulin in response, you become more sensitive to insulin, which, in turn, leads to stabilized blood sugar levels and fewer crashes and spikes. All of this makes you feel more clear-headed and full of energy.

Promotes an Anti-inflammatory Response

We discussed previously how chronic inflammation is related to an increased risk of developing chronic diseases such as diabetes, arthritis, and heart disease.

However, what you might not know is that when you fast for 12 hours a day for a month, it lowers the inflammatory markers in your body. This helps in keeping your body in shape overall.

Protects Your Heart

When we talk about risk factors related to heart disease, high cholesterol plays a big part. In a small study conducted in 2010 (Bhutani et al., 2010), fasting on alternate days drastically reduced LDL cholesterol levels by 25 percent and triglycerides by 32 percent. This decrease is good for your heart as well as your arteries. When your heart is working better every cell in your body benefits.

Other studies have shown that if you make fasting a part of your routine, you have less chance of having heart failure when compared to people of similar background and diet who do not use fasting as part of their lifestyle.

Promotes Brain Health

Does fasting keep Alzheimer's disease or general cognitive decline at bay? Well, research conducted on mice suggests that it might have a protective effect on the brain and mental health since fasting helps fight inflammation (Mattson & Arumugam, 2018). Because it increases heart health, it also means more oxygenated blood is getting to the brain and associated tissues.

Gains at the Gym

If you're concerned that fasting will not enable you to perform well at the gym or you won't be able to reap the benefits of your exercise program, you need to know that people following fasting programs can still gain lean muscle, lose extra fat, and enhance their performance (Tinsley et al., 2019). You may have to adjust your exercise program to focus more on low-impact cardio and more weight work, but there's no reason you can't or won't continue to improve in this area too.

Protects Against Depression

Fasting has an antidepressant effect, thanks to its ability to produce neurotransmitters such as serotonin and make endogenous opioids available to your brain. That sounds like a mouthful, but put simply, it means that the body releases more natural chemicals that improve your mood and regulate mood swings. Fasting along with restricting calories during non-fasting periods can lead to a reduction in negative emotions such as anger and tension and boost feelings of relaxation.

May Reduce the Risk of Developing Cancer

Here's a disclosure: experts are still learning a lot about the relationship between cancer and fasting. However, animal studies suggest that fasting periodically has an anti-cancer effect (Nencioni et al., 2018).

The research also suggests that fasting makes cancer therapies such as chemotherapy more effective.

Helps You Live Longer

Fasting helps your cells to repair themselves, which can be the reason why it's related to a lowered risk of developing chronic diseases, including cardiovascular and metabolic diseases. It allows you to have better health overall and contributes to a longer life.

So, will limiting your food intake help you live to 100? Well, I can't guarantee you that. But I can tell you that in a study of rats (Goodrick et al., 1982), those that fasted every other day aged at a comparatively slower rate and lived about 83 percent longer than the ones who did not fast. Now, that's something!

Different Fasting Diets and How to Choose the Best One for You

Fasting is not just a scientifically proven way of managing your weight. Different types of fasting diets allow your body to get rid of cellular waste and enhance your mood. From improving your memory to lowering your risk of potential disease, you can get many benefits from fasting.

Fasting fits into any kind of diet, but if you wish to structure it for the best results, you have several options to choose from. Depending on your health goals, current health levels, and eating habits, you will find the style that will fit into your routine.

What are Fasting Diets?

When it comes to fasting diets, there is no one diet that will suit everyone. These diets generally give a specific period of time when you eat, and is often focused on specialized food groups, followed by times that you go without food or liquids that contain calories.

With this diet, you might want to skip breakfast several times a week, or you might want to limit your food eating window daily. It all depends on what works best for you.

General Rules for all Types of Fasting Diets

Make sure that you keep in mind the following things when you take up any fasting diet.

- Keep yourself fully hydrated by maintaining regular water intake. When you're fasting, you will probably need to drink more water than you usually do.
- Cutting down on all carbohydrates and consuming the right fats in your eating window can help you to avoid blood sugar crashes that you might otherwise experience during your fasting period. You can try experimenting with different fasting diets and see how your body responds and how you feel about them.
- Stock up on your go-to drinks that will help carry you through your fasting. Unless you are on a strict water-only diet, you can sip on your favorite plain tea, lemon water, or milk-free coffee.

- If you wish to exercise, make sure that you time your eating window around your exercise or workout sessions. Many people prefer hitting the gym when they are abstaining from food, but others find this makes them lightheaded or nauseous. Experiment to find what works best for you and your body.
- On the days when you're not fasting, make sure to have drinks and snacks at the ready for when you feel your energy levels going down. Low-carb options that are high in healthy fat are ideal choices.
- When you break the fast, be sure to break it well. The best fasting diet foods include fruits, vegetables, lean grass-fed meats, and quality fats to enhance maximum nutrient intake in your body.

Types of Fasting Diets

Now that know what you should keep in mind when you're on a fasting diet, let's go through the different kinds of plans that you can try.

16:8 Fasting Diet

The 16:8 fasting diet is among the most popular and is perfect for anyone who is new to the world of fasting.

- The 16:8 fasting plan is an intermittent diet in which you limit consuming food to one eight-hour window daily, generally between noon and 8 p.m.
- To get the best results, limit your carbs at dinner during your eating window and stay hydrated

during the day with lots of water. Drinks with no calories, such as herbal teas, coffee, and lemon water are all allowable at any time with this diet. Some herbal teas, such as cinnamon and dandelion root have been found to help suppress appetite and can make fasting easier.

- Once you adapt to a 16-hour fast, you can try an 18-hour fast with a six-hour eating window to avail yourself of even more benefits of intermittent fasting.

The basic 16:8 structure is not meant to restrict your food choices during your eating window. But consuming a low-carb diet rich in fruits, vegetables, and lean meats will help keep your blood sugar levels in check. This will make it easier for you to avoid feeling grumpy during the fasting hours, which can be a drawback of fasting. Also, a low-carb diet makes it simpler for you to get into the process of ketosis, which offers you an added advantage to suppress your appetite.

5:2 Fasting Diet

Studies have suggested that the 5:2 fasting diet leads to weight loss and improves insulin resistance in your body, which reduces your risk of developing type-2 diabetes when compared to just restricting the calories. The principles of the 5:2 eating plan are as follows:

- Eat a reasonable diet five days a week. For the other two days of the week, limit your intake strictly to a maximum of 500-600 calories.

- Have three smaller meals or two larger meals on your calorie-restricted days.
- If you are looking to curb your hunger, try spacing your fasting days between the eating ones.

Eat-Stop-Eat Fasting Diet

The eat-stop-eat fasting diet has you follow your regular healthy eating patterns for most days of the week then fast for 24 hours twice a week between these eating periods. When you fast for 24 hours twice a week, you create a calorie deficit in your body and kick-start the ketosis process. However, 24 hours is a long period for your body to go without food. If you're interested in this type of eating pattern, it's best to consult with your nutritionist or doctor to be sure your body will react well to it. Many people suffer from headaches or mood swings if they fast for extended periods, so this may be a plan you need to work up to gradually. The guidelines for the eat-stop-eat fasting diet are:

- Fast for 24 hours twice a week on non-consecutive days and eat normally for the rest of the days.
- Consume nutrition-rich foods in your eating days and don't binge your calories.
- You can choose to eat something each day by spacing out your 24-hour fasting period. For instance, try eating at 7:00 a.m. on a Friday, start your fast at 8:00 a.m. and start eating again after 8:00 a.m. on Saturday.
- Stay hydrated. You can consume water and other non-calorie bearing drinks such as herbal teas, lemon water, or coffee, although caffeinated beverages should be limited.

4:3 Fasting Diet, or Alternate-Day Fasting

In the 4:3 fasting diet plan, you eat less than 500 calories every other day – those are your fast days. However, with so many fasting days, it can become quite tricky to stick to your schedule. Research suggests that this diet can lead you to feeling irritated and hungry, which may prevent you from maintaining it for a longer duration. However, to stay on track, stay distracted and busy during the fasting days.

- Fast alternate days and eat normally on the other non-fasting days. In a week, you will eat for four days alternatively and fast on the other three. You can also try the opposite, which is fasting for four days and eating for three days.
- On the fasting days, consume no more than 500 calories.
- On non-fasting days, eat a normal, healthy diet without overeating. Stick to fruits, vegetables, whole grains, and lean meats.
- Stay hydrated by drinking ample water, lemon water, and herbal teas.

Warrior Diet

The results of the warrior diet will greatly vary, depending on how much you're willing to reduce your food intake and what you consume during your eating window.

- Fast or eat less than you generally eat for a 20-hour window. Then consume one large meal during an evening eating window of four hours.

- When you are in the fasting window, you can consume small amounts of green leafy veggies or berries, proteins like poached eggs, or zero-calorie liquids such as water or green tea.
- When you choose your evening meal, consume organic, wholesome, and nutrient-rich foods.

One Meal A Day, or OMAD

The One Meal A Day diet offers you all the benefits of fasting while simplifying your overall approach and schedule. Because of its very restrictive nature, it's more difficult to follow, so it may not be the best fasting diet to begin with and should not be maintained for too long. Also, it's not for children, the elderly, those who have suffered from eating disorders, or those who are pregnant.

- Fast for 23 hours and consume your daily calories in your one-hour window.
- To give your body enough time to eat socially and to ensure you can digest your food before you sleep, consider eating between 4 p.m. and 7 p.m. daily.
- When you sit to eat, make sure that you consume a nutritional and balanced meal.

Impromptu Meal Skipping

This diet is the perfect option for someone who wants to have complete flexibility, since it relies on an intuitive approach to eating.

- Don't eat when you don't feel hungry.

- When you eat, opt for your normal, healthy diet.
- Stay hydrated.
- To keep your weight healthy and stable, your blood sugar levels steady, and extend the fasting window, consume a diet that has fewer carbs and more high quality-fats in your non-fasting windows.

How to Find the Best Fasting Diet for You

You need to make sure that you consult with your health-care professional before you try a fasting diet. Fasting is not for people who possess a history of eating disorders, have some chronic diseases or imbalances, or have a history of disordered eating patterns.

Fasting might seem difficult in the beginning, especially when you haven't tried this type of eating schedule before. But when you follow the right fasting diet, you can control your eating habits and gain the maximum advantages. Just like any other kind of healthy eating, you will want to experiment to find what version of this diet works for you the best and what your body will accept most readily. Start by having a larger window, such as 16:8, as it will be easier for you to start with, and then you can gradually step into the longer fasting windows.

Downsides of a Fasting Diet

Fasting diets certainly are popular, and studies have proven the potential benefits. But there are some issues that should be considered and may be downsides to trying this kind of diet.

- The biggest drawback of fasting is that people are not prepared to transition into consuming a healthy diet once the fasting window is closed. When they stop the extreme calorie deficit they overeat and choose the wrong kinds of foods. When this happens the benefits of the fast are lost.
- When fasting goes on too long or isn't appropriately balanced it may lead to losing muscle instead of fat, decreased metabolic rate, headaches, and acidosis.
- Long-term fasting and fasting diets are generally not recommended for children, the elderly, or pregnant people.

When done moderately, fasting promotes weight loss as long as you transition into eating healthy food that is low or moderate in carbs afterward.

What are the Health Risks of Fasting Diets?

Although a lot more research still needs to be carried out in order to understand the long-term benefits as well as the risks of fasting diets, the short-term risks should not be ignored. These include fatigue, irritability, and headaches. The electrolytes in your body get disrupted when you are fasting, but this can be monitored through blood tests, if necessary.

- If you're considering a detox or fasting diet, you need to first consult with your doctor.
- If you're on medications for diabetes or blood pressure, you might need to reduce your medicines

when you are fasting. Also, diabetics may experience fluctuating blood sugar levels.

Key Takeaways

Science suggests that fasting may be associated with a great number of health benefits, including regulation of your blood sugar levels, reducing weight, and keeping your body in overall good condition. There are several good reasons to try it out, just make sure that you consult with your doctor before you begin.

We have talked about some of the different ways in which you can detox and diets that may be used as part of detoxing. Now let's look at how you can detox safely and what precautions you need to take before, during, and after your detox.

9

Before, During, and After Detox

I f you have ever thought of trying out a detox diet, there are several things that you need to consider before, during, and after.

A healthy detox plan is one that aims to enhance the natural detoxification processes of your body by changing your eating habits. Detox diets may result in weight loss, but they are not meant for weight loss specifically.

Make sure that you don't fall into the trap of following a plan that suggests you stop eating or drinking altogether to cleanse your system. That's definitely not how a healthy detox diet works.

When you're not feeding your body anything at all, your metabolism takes it as a signal that it will not be getting any of the nutrition it needs to function. It thinks it's starving, and it's right! As a result, your body will retain water and fat to protect itself and may even feed on your lean muscle mass. This isn't the goal. Detoxification is about helping your body to remove toxins and be healthier, not to shut your systems down.

Why is it Crucial to Detox Regularly?

If you're wondering why you need to detox on a regular basis, let me tell you the truth. Because of the things we eat, drink, breathe in, and generally encounter in our daily lives, we are all toxic; but some of us are more toxic than others.

If you're healthy, the natural detoxification of your body is running smoothly. But if you're consuming or absorbing a lot of toxins, then the mechanism for detoxification in your liver can become sluggish.

In the end, certain toxins create havoc in your body by sticking around. They make you feel tired, sick, and fat — or what you might call "I feel like crap" syndrome.

In a perfect world, we would all be free of toxins. But in reality, with our poor diets and modern lifestyles, everyone suffers from some toxicity. From the air we inhale to the food we consume to the chemicals we are exposed to in our daily routines, it's pretty simple for toxins to build up in our bodies. For this reason, it's important to detoxify our bodies on a regular basis.

How Often Should You Detox and For How Long is a Detox Effective?

- Before you start your detox journey, make sure that it's a good time of the year for you to stick with it.

For example, you might want to consider starting in the spring when there are fewer holidays.

- Choose a time that you're not pregnant or recovering from any illnesses.
- When you're detoxing, lighten your exercise routine since you have fewer calories to burn.
- Try for two detoxes every year, so you have about six months between them.
- You might experience short-term weight loss during detox, but don't expect it to stay that way. Detoxes are not meant for weight loss unless you are targeting gas and bloating.
- There's a chance that you will feel worse in the beginning of your detox before you start to feel better. Many people complain about feeling grumpy or sluggish since they don't get to eat what they're generally used to, and they might be giving up caffeine too. Stick to your plan!
- Your detox journey should only last for a few days to one month, and no longer until the next detox period.

The Biggest Offender You Need to Detoxify From

One of the biggest diet offenders that we might not consider a toxin is sugar. Sugar in all its different forms is the primary cause of our obesity epidemic. It's related to most of the chronic diseases that plague us and our economy, and in the rest of the world too.

If you're addicted to sugar and flour (which gets broken down to sugar in the body when digested), it's not considered an emotional eating disorder. It is, in fact, a biological disorder, which is driven by our neurotransmitters and hormones that fuel carb and sugar cravings, and ultimately leads to uncontrolled overeating. This is the reason about 70 percent of Americans, including 40 percent of kids, are overweight.

Part of the problem is that we are born with the innate understanding that most sweet foods are safe to eat and most bitter foods are poisonous or not safe to eat. In times when processed sugars were not readily available, this biological training had an important function. At that time, the natural attraction to sweet foods didn't lead to as many problems because the available items were naturally sweet like fruits, vegetables, and honey. However, we live in a time when sugar and refined carbs are abundant, fast, and inexpensive, so we can't trust our natural urges about what we should eat to maintain healthy bodies.

We often blame people for being sick and overweight. But it's not entirely their fault. The junk food industry has hijacked our brains, taste buds, and hormones so that we keep eating junk food (particularly refined sugar, salt and fat), but in reality all our body is doing is craving natural food. Next time you crave some junk food, try having a fresh, crisp apple and see if the craving is still there afterwards.

How to Begin Your Healthy Detox Journey

If you're ready to begin your detox journey, start by visiting your doctor and discussing your plan and symptoms with them. You may think that your body is just loaded with toxins (which is probably true), but it can also be something more severe than that. So, it's vital that you get assessed before starting detox. Your doctor will be able to recommend the food and lifestyle changes that are the healthiest for you and your body.

Know Your Body Well

Only you know what happens to your body in the course of a normal day. If you have a demanding schedule or intense workout sessions, you may have to adjust these habits while you are detoxing, based on how you're feeling. Once you're on your diet, make sure that you listen to and understand your body and the signals it sends. Biologically and psychologically, many people do not react well to detox, so you might need to try several different options over time to find out which one works best with your body. Know the difference between annoyances that you may have to work through and when your body is really in distress.

Make a Plan

Once you've talked to your doctor, decide on a plan. We've talked about several detox diet options in this book. Look for an option that suits your current health and your lifestyle, then consider what things you need to do in preparation to start. It can help to write out your menus for a shopping trip so you can have everything on hand before you start. You don't want to give yourself any excuses to give up on your diet, and that means being prepared to commit to see the detox through, focusing on the positive benefits you will receive.

Elements of a Solid Detox Plan

There are several commercial detox plans and programs that you may find. Beware that many are extremely high in sugars and too low in good fats. Good fats will help you feel full and give your body necessary fatty acids to detox properly. I recommend that you consume quality fats when you are on your detox diet. These kinds of fats are found in organic chicken, eggs, olive oil, coconut oil, coconut butter, grass-fed beef, raw nuts and seeds, and low-mercury fish like salmon.

The Biggest Mistake People Make While Detoxing

The biggest mistake people frequently make when they are detoxing is thinking, "Oh, I feel so good now, I can go back to whatever I was doing before."

Consider the detox diet to be a chance for you to reconnect with your body and choose how you wish to feel and live. Detoxing shouldn't be permission to follow an unhealthy lifestyle when you aren't on your detox diet, but it should be a starting point for a much healthier lifestyle overall.

How to Optimize Detoxification

If you want to have optimized detoxification, consider these things:

- Consume whole, real, fresh, and unprocessed foods that are rich in protein, healthy fats, fiber, and antioxidants.

- Consider detox that eliminates foods that are most commonly associated with allergies or intolerances.
- Bacterial overgrowth or infections can prevent your gut from functioning properly. Talk to your doctor if you notice these or any other issues.
- Replenish the digestive enzymes in your body by eating unsweetened yogurt or kefir. If you don't have the required digestive enzymes in your body, the food you eat cannot get converted to the raw material that your body needs to function. You can also consider taking broad-spectrum digestive enzymes with your meals.
- Be sure to eat enough good fats in your diet and take omega-3 supplements. This will ease any gut inflammation.
- Rebuild the friendly bacteria in your gut by taking probiotic supplements in your diet. These supplements will help to rebuild the healthy gut bacteria that are crucial for your health.
- Take care of the gut lining by consuming nutrients that promote healthy function, like zinc and glutamine.
- Stay hydrated and exercise to keep your body working it's best and flush out toxins.

Have a Support Network

When you're planning your detox diet, talk it over with friends or family that you trust to have your best interests at heart and to give you the support you need. You may want someone to check in with every day or need help removing tempting treats and foods from your house if you're avoiding them during your detox. Exercising is often more effective with a partner, and it's easier to continue to share meals with friends if they know your dietary requirements. Look for support from those who can help you make your detox journey in a positive fashion.

Prepare Your Mind Well

When you start your detox journey with a calm mind, it will help you stay focused and motivated to finish the program. If you lack motivation and a positive state of mind, make a list of the things that you will do once you have succeeded in your journey. List the reasons why you started and what you hope to gain, and it will add to the impetus you need to finish!

Plan for What Happens After Your Detox

When you opt for a detox program, you've already made a great decision toward improving your health.

It's a misconception that once your detox is over, you will say no to all other temptations. But even when you've successfully completed your detox diet, you can still have cravings.

Be prepared with a plan for how you will eat and what healthy lifestyle changes you will carry with you into the rest of your life. Look at your detox as a starting place to a healthier you. If you remove sweets from your house before detoxing, don't bring them back in. If you create a good habit to exercise every morning, keep your schedule clear and keep the exercise. Make the commitment to yourself to continue the healthy journey you have begun.

Key Takeaways

Opting for a detox diet can be a life-changing decision that will lead to a better future. Make plans to make your detox healthy and effective and a starting place for a healthier you.

Consult A Doctor If

Since the detox diet is meant to get rid of the toxins in your body, it allows the consumption of only organic and natural foods and a lot of fluids to help make the process of elimination easier. However, there can be some inadequacies you will have to address to keep yourself healthy.

Generally, detox diets are low in calories and extremely high in natural laxatives (like the fiber in the foods you eat) as well as diuretics. If you don't plan your detox and implement it correctly, it can be harmful to your body.

- The ideal caloric intake for an adult on a daily basis is around 2000 for women and 2500 for men, depending on your level of activity. When your body receives less than the minimum requirement for too long, it can stop or slow the production of the growth hormone. This can result in reduced levels of thyroid hormones and insulin, among others, which results in changes to your body's metabolism and hormonal imbalances.

- Restricting calories leads to nutritional deficiencies. Several detox diets require elimination of specific foods, such as milk, which is a key source of calcium. This could lead to a calcium deficiency in your body. For this reason, you might want to consider a good quality daily multivitamin when you're detoxing.
- When your body is deficient in nutrients, it leads to a weaker immune system. This can be offset by choosing lemon water and other citrus foods that feed your immune system.
- When you restrict calories severely, your body can go into starvation mode and reduce its metabolism, making it difficult for you to lose weight.
- When planning a fasting diet, keep in mind that when you fast for longer periods, it can lead to muscle breakdown. Weight loss here occurs due to the loss of muscles and not fat.
- Since detox diets contain a lot of natural diuretics and laxatives, they can lead to mineral deficiencies in your body along with fatigue, dizziness, headaches, and nausea. The healthy gut bacteria that you need may also get flushed out of your system, leading to gastrointestinal problems.

Preparing for Detox

Once you have decided to participate in a period of detoxing there are a few things you can do to prepare your body and ease into the plan.

- Cut back on alcohol, sugar, excess soda, caffeine, processed foods, and sugar substitutes. This keeps you from going "cold turkey" when your detox begins.
- Get used to giving your body the nutrient-rich foods it needs so it can use these nutrients to perform its daily functions. Increase the number of fruits and vegetables you eat each day. Try new things and stock up on the healthy foods that you like and some you've never tried before. If you increase the fiber in your diet before you begin your detox you will not have sudden issues with gas or diarrhea brought on by suddenly increasing your fiber intake.
- Start drinking more water. When you first increase your water consumption, you'll find you have to go to the bathroom more often than usual as your body releases retained water. This improves as your body becomes accustomed to being properly hydrated, so start early.

Safety of Detoxing

There are no federal guidelines for detoxing or detox programs. The U.S. Federal Trade Commission (FTC) and Food and Drug Administration (FDA) have taken strict action against companies selling cleansing or detoxing products that (1) contain any illegal or potentially harmful ingredients; (2) are marketed with false claims that they can treat any specific diseases; or (3) in the case of medical devices for cleansing colons, were marketed for unapproved uses. Beyond this, it's up to you to work with your doctor and do your research so you can choose a detox diet that will be beneficial to your health situation.

When You Should Contact a Doctor

If you begin a full-body detox and start to feel unwell or experience symptoms like fatigue, vomiting, fever, or diarrhea, then stop the detox right away and consult your doctor.

Final Things to Consider

A full-body detox helps your body to eliminate toxins. Some detoxes recommend you make drastic changes in your diet and lifestyle, while others include products that contain laxatives. These detoxes can be dangerous to your health.

Do your research and choose a detox diet that has a natural, balanced approach. A good detox is an opportunity to start healthy habits which can last a lifetime, like eating more vegetables and fruits, drinking more water, and stopping smoking or drinking.

I wish you all the success with your detoxing journey!

Thank you for taking the time to read Why We Need to Detox. I have thoroughly enjoyed the experience of writing it and I sincerely hope you enjoyed reading it. I would be very grateful if you could leave me a review on Amazon or at **www.magletpublishing.com** to help others realize the benefits of having a body detox every now and again. Just scan the QR code below.

If you'd like to download a free Meal Planner template to help you keep track of what you are going to eat, head over to: www.magletpublishing.com/mealplanner

Other books in the Things We Need To Do series:

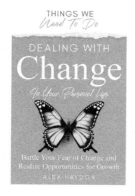
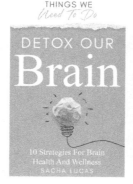
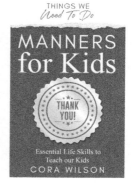

References

Bhutani, S., Klempel, M. C., Berger, R. A., & Varady, K. A. (2010). Improvements in coronary heart disease risk indicators by alternate-day fasting involve adipose tissue modulations. Obesity, 18(11), 2152–2159. https://doi.org/10.1038/oby.2010.54

Bjarnadottir, A. (2019, January 10). Do detox diets and cleanses really work? Healthline. https://www.healthline.com/nutrition/detox-diets-101#toxins

Budgen, O. (2018, November 14). How to support your detox pathways naturally. Olivia Budgen. https://oliviabudgen.com/how-to-support-your-detox-pathways-naturally/

Gaudreau, S. (2019, November 2). Demystifying detox: Tips for supporting your elimination pathways. Steph Gaudreau. https://www.stephgaudreau.com/demystifying-detox-supporting-elimination-pathways/

GiveHer5, T. (2019, April 22). How to detox on your period. A Period Blog. https://www.giveher5.org/blog/2019/04/22/how-to-detox-on-your-period/

Goodrick, C. L., Ingram, D. K., Reynolds, M. A., Freeman, J. R., & Cider, N. L. (1982). Effects of intermittent feeding upon growth and life span in rats. Gerontology, 28(4), 233–241. https://doi.org/10.1159/000212538

Mattson, M. P., & Arumugam, T. V. (2018). Hallmarks of brain aging: Adaptive and pathological modification by metabolic states. Cell Metabolism, 27(6), 1176–1199. https://doi.org/10.1016/j.cmet.2018.05.011

Metrus, L. (2015, February 4). 7-Day detox plan to kick-start your

References

metabolism. HealthyWomen. https://www.healthywomen.org/content/blog-entry/7-day-detox-plan-kick-start-your-metabolism

Nencioni, A., Caffa, I., Cortellino, S., & Longo, V. D. (2018). Fasting and cancer: molecular mechanisms and clinical application. Nature Reviews. Cancer, 18(11), 707–719. https://doi.org/10.1038/s41568-018-0061-0

Tinsley, G. M., & La Bounty, P. M. (2015). Effects of intermittent fasting on body composition and clinical health markers in humans. Nutrition Reviews, 73(10), 661–674. https://doi.org/10.1093/nutrit/nuv041

Tinsley, G. M., Moore, M. L., Graybeal, A. J., Paoli, A., Kim, Y., Gonzales, J. U., Harry, J. R., VanDusseldorp, T. A., Kennedy, D. N., & Cruz, M. R. (2019). Time-restricted feeding plus resistance training in active females: A randomized trial. The American Journal of Clinical Nutrition, 110(3), 628–640. https://doi.org/10.1093/ajcn/nqz126

Watts, Dr. T., & Davidson, Dr. J. (2019, December 30). Drainage 101: Why it's the first step in your detox journey - Microbe FormulasTM. Microbeformulas.com. https://microbeformulas.com/blogs/microbe-formulas/drainage-101-why-it-s-the-first-step-in-your-detox-journey

What's the difference between a detox and cleanse? (2020, June 2). Nourished. https://nourished.com/whats-the-difference-between-a-detox-and-cleanse/

Wroe, M. (2019, March 1). Detox: Let's get our facts straight. St. Jude Wellness Center. http://stjudewellnesscenter.org/2019/03/01/detox-lets-get-our-facts-straight/

Author Bio

My name is Sacha Lucas, and I am passionate about helping others to achieve the level of happiness that I have found through detoxing and decluttering.

I was struggling through life in my early 30s, stressed, overwhelmed, and just completely lost. Then I stopped for a moment, focused on my health and found my way back. I have also wrestled for about two decades with an autoimmune disorder. This disorder and the related stress brought with them gut inflammation leading to pain and irritation that affects my home and work life. It's hard to accomplish anything at all—much less be a great mother and spouse—when you're in pain! But in the last four years, I have found a solution to this irritation and pain by controlling my diet and regularly detoxing.

I am passionate about guiding people through the same process by helping them rebalance their body by giving it a well-earned rest though detoxing.